Thriving in a Relationship When You Have Chronic Illness

Navigate Challenges & Keep Your Relationship Strong Using Acceptance & Commitment Therapy

Lisa Gray, LMFT

New Harbinger Publications, Inc.

Publisher's Note

This publication is designed to provide accurate and authoritative information in regard to the subject matter covered. It is sold with the understanding that the publisher is not engaged in rendering psychological, financial, legal, or other professional services. If expert assistance or counseling is needed, the services of a competent professional should be sought.

NEW HARBINGER PUBLICATIONS is a registered trademark of New Harbinger Publications, Inc.

New Harbinger Publications is an employee-owned company.

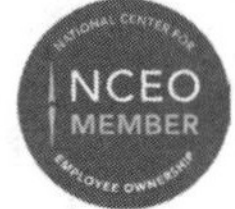

New Harbinger Publications, Inc.
5720 Shattuck Avenue
Oakland, CA 94609
www.newharbinger.com

Cover design by Amy Shoup

Acquired by Georgia Kolias

Edited by Kristi Hein

Library of Congress Cataloging-in-Publication Data on file

MIX
Paper | Supporting responsible forestry
FSC® C008955
FSC www.fsc.org

Printed in the United States of America

27 26 25

10 9 8 7 6 5 4 3 2 1 First Printing

"This book doesn't shy away from the challenges that health issues bring to an intimate relationship, but it doesn't surrender to them either. With deep compassion and clarity, Lisa Gray shows how—with courage, care, and the right support—couples can not only stay connected but use these challenges as a pathway to deeper emotional intimacy."

—**Mali Apple** and **Joe Dunn**, authors of *The Soulmate Experience* and *Wild Monogamy*

"*Thriving in a Relationship When You Have Chronic Illness* is a compassionate, easy-to-follow resource for couples facing unique relational challenges. It offers clear tools, realistic options, and thoughtful guidance on intimacy, communication, and family impact—topics too often ignored. As a therapist, I appreciate how it brings validation and practical support to those seeking connection and understanding in the midst of chronic illness."

—**Michelle Engblom-Deglmann, PhD, LMFT,** tenured professor of counseling at George Fox University, and author of *The Heart of Counseling*

"For those suffering from chronic illnesses and their partners, Lisa Gray has assembled a lovely and wise book using the principles of acceptance and commitment therapy (ACT) to help couples navigate strains and struggles with care and appreciation for one another. The exercises and vignettes within are clear and well organized, and readers will discover Lisa's voice to be one of warmth and compassion emerging from her own personal experiences with chronic illness and her clinical expertise."

—**Scott Spradlin, LPC, LMAC,** author of *Don't Let Your Emotions Run Your Life*, and codirector of Wichita DBT at NorthStar Therapy

"*Thriving in a Relationship When You Have Chronic Illness* is a compassionate, practical guide that brings clarity, empathy, and hope to a deeply challenging experience. Lisa Gray beautifully weaves 'well partner' and 'sick partner' perspectives with mindful, actionable tools. A must-read for anyone navigating love in the context of illness."

—**Shayna Kaufmann, PhD**, psychologist, mindfulness teacher, and author of *Embrace the Middle*

"This book is a lifeline for couples facing chronic illness—one I wish I'd had when I went through it myself. It's a must-read, filled with hope and compassion, for the millions navigating a medical merry-go-round."

—**Dana Parish**, coauthor of *Chronic*

Contents

	A Note to the Chronically Ill	iv
	Foreword	v
	Introduction	1
Chapter 1	Shock and Denial Phase	11
Chapter 2	Tools for Shock and Denial	23
Chapter 3	Anger Phase	35
Chapter 4	Tools for the Anger Phase	47
Chapter 5	Bargaining Phase	59
Chapter 6	Tools for the Bargaining Phase	71
Chapter 7	Depression Phase	83
Chapter 8	Tools for the Depression Phase	95
Chapter 9	Testing and Acceptance	107
Chapter 10	Tools for Testing and Acceptance	119
Chapter 11	Going Forward	131
	Acknowledgments	136
	Resources	137
	References	138

A Note to the Chronically Ill

I've often heard that it's nearly impossible to read a "dense" book when you suffer with the fatigue and brain fog of chronic illness—and having experienced this myself, I agree. On the other hand, there are days and periods of clarity, and I don't want to leave out powerful information that could be helpful.

For these reasons, I've included "What You Will Learn in This Chapter" bullet points at the beginning of every grief stage chapter so you can determine whether that chapter can help you right now. If reading an entire chapter isn't possible for you, jump to the "Chapter Summary" bullet points at the end of each chapter.

If you're going through a low period or flare-up, I suggest you look only for the chapters that apply to where you are right now. You don't have to read this book in order. In the grief stage chapter, read the "What You Will Learn" and "Summary" points. In the tools chapter, choose one (just one!) exercise for the ill partner and focus on trying to practice that skill.

Foreword

When Lisa asked me to write this foreword, I was so grateful to know this book would soon be born. Having traversed the rugged terrain of chronic illness myself, while trying to maintain a healthy relationship, I know intimately the challenges this book addresses. In my memoir *Brave New Medicine*, I chronicled my own journey as a doctor, mother, and partner through mysterious symptoms, and the profound isolation that chronic illness can bring. My husband would return home flushed with the energy of his workday, while I remained in the same spot he'd left me that morning, too exhausted to shower. We moved through this period differently—him moving forward at full speed, and my needing to pause and go deeper. Moving in different directions, I wondered, Can we stay together, let alone in a healthy way or not? I couldn't see that he was suffering as much as I was, but differently. A roadmap like Lisa has created in these pages would've been a guiding light in those dark days.

When chronic illness enters a relationship, it doesn't just affect the person who's sick. It barges in like an uninvited third party who fundamentally alters the partnership, reshaping dynamics in ways neither person is prepared to navigate. Lisa knows this both as a therapist who works with people living with chronic pain, and firsthand, as someone who has lived through chronic illness. The dreams you shared, the activities that connected you, even your most intimate moments—everything turns on its side and inside-out. Without practical tools, many couples find themselves drifting apart precisely when they need each other the most.

Throughout my career, I've witnessed the contrast between couples who navigate illness with grace and compassion, often growing through the experience, and those who crumble under the weight of unforeseen changes. This isn't a judgment, but an observation that highlights a crucial truth. The difference often boils down to having accessible tools, resources, and support. With the six-step guide Lisa offers here, this period of trial can become one of profound growth and deepened compassion—for yourself, your partner, or another relationship.

A fundamental point that Lisa recognizes is how both partners are experiencing their own form of grief, often in different ways and at different times. Through a thoughtful application of Acceptance and Commitment Therapy principles (ACT), she offers concrete strategies for each phase of this journey. I particularly appreciate her emphasis on values. When illness strips away so much of what defined your life together, reconnecting with your core values can illuminate a path forward with regard to time and money that honors what matters to both of you. This wasn't intuitive for me—I spent too long trying to return to the person I was before illness struck, rather than discovering who I could be in the present moment.

Lisa also points out that this journey isn't linear. Though separate, your two journeys are also inseparable. She offers a way to protect and even deepen your bond. So whether you're the partner who's facing the health challenge or the partner who remains well, and whether you're newly diagnosed or years into this journey, let the methods of this book accompany and support you.

This book is a golden resource for patients and healthcare professionals alike. As your inner and outer landscapes evolve, return to these pages whenever you need guidance. Because just as chronic illness doesn't happen in isolation, neither does healing. Know that your relationship can survive this. More so, it can thrive.

—*Cynthia Li, MD*
Physician and author

Introduction

On the day we get married or otherwise commit to one another, we have many grand dreams for our lives. Most of us imagine days filled with love and sunshine, successful careers, perhaps children, with these joys continuing until we are side by side on the porch rocking chairs.

I don't need to tell you how often these dreams don't come true, for a variety of reasons. But perhaps one of the most unanticipated forms of loss happens when one partner contracts an unexpected chronic illness. I'm not sure why it's so unexpected, because according to the National Health Council, 133 million Americans—40 percent of the population—have at least one chronic illness (American Hospital Association 2007). But we rarely anticipate that will be part of our story.

Many kinds of illnesses can impact our relationships, including mental illnesses or terminal illnesses. Devastating as these may be in their own right, they're not the subject of this book, although you may still be able to glean some useful information. This book addresses the types of chronic conditions that affect one partner's ability to physically function and will affect the couple and their dynamics going forward, but which have no cure and cannot be expected to significantly change. There are no curative treatments for the conditions, nor will they necessarily lead to loss of life. Some examples are autoimmune and immune diseases, fatigue, chronic migraines, chronic non-life-threatening heart or respiratory issues, diabetes, traumatic brain injury, and chronic pain without an organic cause. There are many others, and the global COVID pandemic has created a few more.

From the moment symptoms begin, the couple's experiences start to diverge. One partner faces the loss of functionality and lifestyle to some degree, and the other partner faces the loss of the partnership they thought they chose. They now have many hurdles to overcome, together and individually. In addition, whatever patterns of interacting or issues were already present in the relationship become amplified to the nth degree.

It's my hope to help partners navigate these changes without losing a relationship they can define as intimate and satisfying. It will not be the same partnership you had prior to the onset of symptoms, but it can still be a very satisfying one.

In this book I use the words "couple," "relationship," and "partnership" interchangeably; the experiences in this book can apply to any variety of intimate relationship—dating, married, cohabitating, nonmonogamous, and so on. The dynamics I describe usually refer to a dyad (two people), but they can also be applied to other forms of relationship.

The Stages of Grief for Chronic Illness

Because this journey is a grieving process for both partners, often for different reasons, to frame the problem I've organized this book into the common stages of grief.

I'll guide you through each stage in order—although the stages of grief are better described as a pendulum that we may cycle through, and not necessarily in order or even just once. This "stage" description of grief isn't used as regularly in the therapeutic community as it once was, but I'll use it here because most people have some familiarity with the concepts. At each stage, I'll note what the couple's experience might be, in addition to the differing concerns of well partner and ill partner.

Shock and Denial

Whether the illness's onset is sudden (like chronic pain from an accident or a traumatic brain injury from a fall) or very gradual (like joint pain or mysterious fatigue), the process usually begins with some kind of shock or denial. If there is a sudden onset, usually shock rules the day. How can your lives have changed so dramatically in the blink of an eye? If more gradual, it may take more of a denial form. Surely you can still hike all day Saturday even though you're fatigued without explanation. Or surely your partner can still give you a back rub even though they say their joints are in pain and distress. Often, you're thrown by the ice-cold shower of shock or the slow adjustment of denial seeping into your consciousness until it becomes clear that things will not be the same as they were.

Anger

Next, you're likely to, very appropriately, move on to anger. How dare your life turn out this way? You may be angry at the medical community, which you previously thought could cure what ails you but now realize is set up mainly for acute disease and apparently has no idea what to do with chronic disease. You might be mad at a higher power or the universe for your drawing such a bad hand. And all too often, you begin to be angry at each other, even if that doesn't make any sense. You may have chosen your partner because you both love travel, and now they can't travel. How *dare* they change the narrative like that? Or maybe you're the one who isn't well, and your partner doesn't know how to talk to you about that, or is continuing to do all the fun things you can no longer do, and this leaves you irate. Again, it may not make sense, but there are so many ways that rage can tear our relationships apart at this stage.

Bargaining

Next comes bargaining, or the "if onlys." If only your partner had eaten better, maybe they wouldn't have diabetes. If only you had not fallen off that ladder and injured your brain. If only your partner would eat totally healthy, maybe they wouldn't have diabetes any more. Or if only you would do a certain kind of physical therapy, maybe your brain would work as it used to. Often during this stage you'll try to "do better" or think of actions that could change this new reality. Or maybe you try to make a deal with those higher powers to receive some kind of miracle. And all too often, partners experience this stage differently. One might want to go back to church, while the other is angry at a god they thought was looking out for them. One might be lost in self-recriminations, while the other is ready to accept reality and move on. One might be judging things their partner could have or should have done to stay well, and the ill partner feels that judgment.

Depression

Of course, when none of this bargaining results in any changes, depression is often the result. For one partner, depression means really understanding that they're never going to be well; never going to be the same person, able to do the same things that they did before they got sick. The other partner can also be depressed, realizing that although they're well, they have a commitment to another person who isn't—something that is going to affect the rest of their lives, even though the well partner can still do everything they always could. Both partners may feel isolated in their experience but not able to offer each other comfort. Because many chronic illnesses are invisible and can't be seen by others, you may also suffer great losses or shifts in community. Feeling seen and understood requires that others believe what the ill person reports, and many people (sometimes even our partner) have difficulty doing that.

Testing and Acceptance

Coming out of depression, you enter the phase of testing, which isn't on all published stages of grief conceptualizations, but which I think fits well into this process. In this phase, partners begin to test out different solutions that might help them adjust to this new reality. Some may be solutions that they do together, and some may be separate solutions.

Finally comes the stage of acceptance (more on this word follows)—a full commitment to the new reality and all of the challenges that it presents.

Each stage presents a minefield for partners as they navigate myriad issues, including (but not limited to) communication, shared activities, sex and intimacy, friendships, emotional experiences, roles, support systems, practical considerations, and navigating the medical world. Because each of us looks at these subjects differently, each will have a different way of handling these challenges. These topics are difficult enough for partners when there is *no* extenuating circumstance, but they're excruciating when chronic illness is at play.

Each stage requires a new skill to help you adjust to your new reality. The vehicle that I use to help build the skills you will need is *acceptance and commitment therapy*, or ACT.

ACT Explained

A simple explanation of ACT is that it aims for complete acceptance of your circumstances and all emotions associated with that, paired with committed behaviors that align with your life's values. A main ACT component is the *choice point*—a point in time or circumstance where you choose to move either toward or away from your stated values. So it's important to decide, as we go, not only your individual values but also what you value as a team.

The goal of ACT is "psychological flexibility" (very useful in situations of chronic illness). ACT entails six core processes; we'll discuss one of these for each of the recognized six stages of the grief process. Clearly, real life is not organized in such neat boxes—and in the last chapter I'll help you see how you can mix and match these stages. But it's helpful to use an ACT core process in tandem with each grief stage. If you're a visual person, it might look something like the figure shown here.

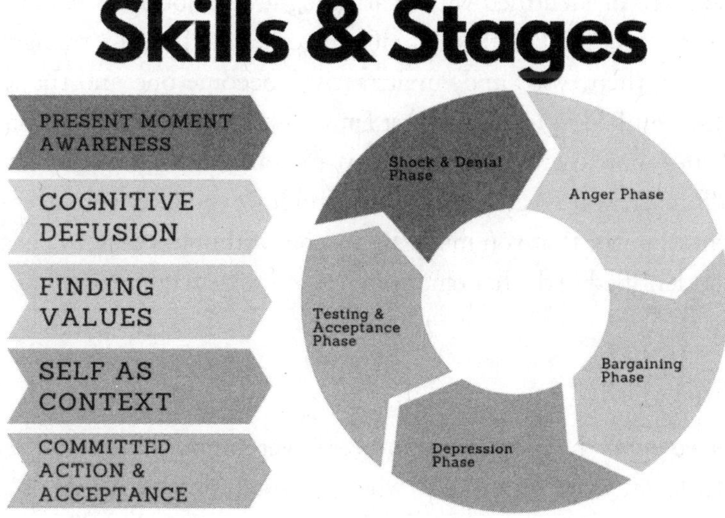

Present Moment Awareness

In the stage of shock and denial, it's useful to learn the ACT core process of *present moment awareness*; more simply, being in the moment. Because this stage contains so many unknowns, you can easily get into what I call "future-tripping"—wildly predicting what might come next. Or, in the case of denial, you may be reluctant to let go of your past self or to align with what is happening now. For each partner, learning to be in the present moment not only lays a foundation for many coming experiences, but also allows for processing only what needs to be processed *now.* It also allows each person, and the partnership, to begin recognizing the power of simply being with themself or each other, in whatever is happening now, instead of what you may *wish* were happening.

Cognitive Defusion

The stage of anger can be particularly frightening, especially for people who haven't experienced strong angry feelings before, or who are very uncomfortable with the emotion of anger. For this stage the skill is *cognitive defusion.* It may seem technical, but we've all experienced it: your mind gets "hooked" on a thought or emotion you're having (kind of like a dog with a really yummy bone) and refuses to let go of it. You become fused or identified with that thought or emotion as real or true when it may not be. For example, if you get hooked on the thought *I'm unattractive*, then "you" and "unattractive" become one and the same. But if you think *How interesting that I'm struggling with the thought that I'm unattractive*, now there's distance between you and the thought. In this stage I'll teach you several skills that can allow you to experience all of the rightful anger that you might be feeling, without necessarily becoming overidentified with that emotion.

Finding Values

As we enter the bargaining phase, it's very important to *find values*, so that you can orient yourself to what is actually true. If you don't know your values, your "if onlys" can spiral out of control, and you'll be lost in recriminations against yourself or your partner. Or, in seeking to make things right by being a better person or searching for a miracle, you could spend a lot of time or money on things that won't solve the problem and may present more relationship issues if you don't know how to align with your value system. Each person will need to develop their own individual values and align those with the values they have as a team, which may be no easy task.

Self-as-Context

The ACT skill for the depression phase of grief is *self-as-context*, which may perplex those not already familiar with the Buddhist concept of the observing self. There's no need to be religious or spiritual here, nor to be familiar with that concept. The observing self is simply understanding that there's a "you" inside that can observe your thoughts and feelings but isn't actually you. Confusing? Here's an example: Let's say that you think *I hate myself for being sick*. There's a part of yourself that is aware that you're just thinking this; that it's simply a thought and that *you* are separate from the thought. This aligns with depression because during this phase, partners will have many hopeless thoughts about a variety of things—the lack of care within the medical system, the things they can no longer do, the things they have lost and so on. Without an observing self, you're at risk for becoming these thoughts and not being able to find your way out of this jungle.

Committed Action

When you do emerge, and you begin to "test" new ideas for life in the context of chronic disease, you need *committed action*. During this phase, you choose to experiment with various ways of thinking and a variety of new behaviors that can build a life of meaning for each partner individually and as a team. You've identified your values; now as you experiment, you can identify certain committed actions you can take in a number of areas that will align with those values and that you can carry forward as you move along. Because you're a partnership, you also need to make sure that your individual committed actions also line up well with the values you've identified as a team.

Acceptance

Finally, you reach acceptance, for which the ACT core process *is* acceptance. Acceptance doesn't mean giving up, and it doesn't mean you approve of how things are. If you're having a strong reaction to this word and feel like throwing this book across the room, I totally get it. Some people use the word "adaptation" instead of acceptance, because how can you accept the unacceptable? I'll use the word "acceptance" in this book, however, because that's a core word used in both the grief process and in ACT, but feel free to consider it "adaptation" if that works better for you. Also try to trust that if you stick with this process, you'll actually arrive there in the end. It really does mean that you've learned to observe your experiences, unhook from unhelpful thoughts and feelings and choose actions that fit in with your values. In this stage, you've accepted, both individually and as a team, that life has changed—but you've also found ways to live this new life, ways that create growth for each person and for the relationship. This isn't an easy road, but I do firmly believe that by using ACT and working through the grieving process, you can get there.

Why I Wrote This Book

After I had my second child in 2005, I felt like I couldn't recover. Neither of my babies was a very good sleeper, so I thought maybe it was just exhaustion from being a new mom. I also contracted MRSA (a staph infection) shortly after, so I thought maybe it was just that. After a couple of years of thinking perhaps it was normal, I started seeking answers to why I didn't feel well. Over the years, I was told everything was normal, multiple times; twice told I had sleep apnea (I didn't); diagnosed with major depression; and told I was just overweight. Finally, eleven years after my quest began, in 2018 I was diagnosed with Ehlers-Danlos syndrome and chronic fatigue syndrome, neither of which have any great treatment options. I'm very thankful that I have a relatively mild version of both disorders, but it still impacts my life in many unanticipated ways. After my own diagnosis—and being close to others with serious diagnoses—I began to specialize in chronic illness and chronic pain. There are some really excellent books on dealing individually with chronic illness—I'm partial to Toni Bernhard's books *How to Be Sick* (2018) and *How to Live Well with Chronic Illness and Chronic Pain* (2015), but I also like Sarah Ramey's book for women specifically, *The Lady's Handbook for Her Mysterious Illness* (2021). However, in terms of books specifically related to how *partners* cope with one partner having a chronic illness, I was not satisfied with anything then available. I have the profoundly lucky experience of having a very patient and selfless partner, but not everyone is as lucky. And it's still been a real adjustment to the life we thought we were signing up for. Because I've had two specialties now in my career—high-conflict relationships and chronic illness and pain—I felt it was only right to pass along what I've learned.

How to Use This Book

Ideally, partners would read this book together, front to back, in the early stages of chronic illness or chronic pain. But honestly, how often is life ideal? If it were, you wouldn't even be *reading* this book! So if you're in the midst of this life upheaval, and upon reading this introduction you feel that you're really entrenched in a later stage or that one of the ACT processes seems particularly helpful for where you are, please go straight to that chapter. You can always head back to the earlier chapters later. This book includes some intentional repetition, since you may not be reading it from front to back.

Similarly, you may not be reading this book together. You may be the well partner (I prefer the term "well partner" to "caregiver"), searching for ways to deal with the change that has come into your relationship unbidden. There'll be sections and exercises for you in each chapter. Regardless of whether or not your ill partner reads this book, it'll be very helpful for you to gain these skills. And similarly, if you're the ill partner, you'll find sections and exercises that you can do even if your partner can't or won't read this book. Learning these skills individually can't help but improve your relationship and will also immensely help with your personal coping.

Throughout this book, I've included "client" stories to dramatize relationship interactions and experiences. Unless otherwise noted, these stories are fictitious and don't represent any people I've worked with in my practice. Any resemblance to real clients is purely unintentional and not representative of our actual work.

As I've said, grief and its stages just refuse to cooperate in being organized and linear. So even if you do read this book from front to back, you may later find yourself coming back to an earlier stage and needing to read and practice those ACT processes all over again. You aren't doing it wrong; this is just the nature of grief and loss.

I cannot promise you good physical health. There may never be treatments for whatever you're struggling with; there may be times of flare-ups and times of remission. But I *can* promise that you don't have to suffer psychologically or relationally, and I can show you how. Let's jump in and learn to have a satisfying relationship even with the cards you've been dealt.

Chapter 1

Shock and Denial Phase

What You Will Learn in This Chapter:

- Chronic illness can appear suddenly or gradually.
- Sudden-onset chronic illness usually creates a shock reaction, while gradual chronic illness sometimes creates a denial reaction.
- Communication is key as you try to figure out what you're feeling.
- Onset of illness can disrupt shared activity, intimacy, and friendships.
- The ACT skill to cope with shock and denial is learning to be present in the current moment with whatever is happening and whatever you're feeling.

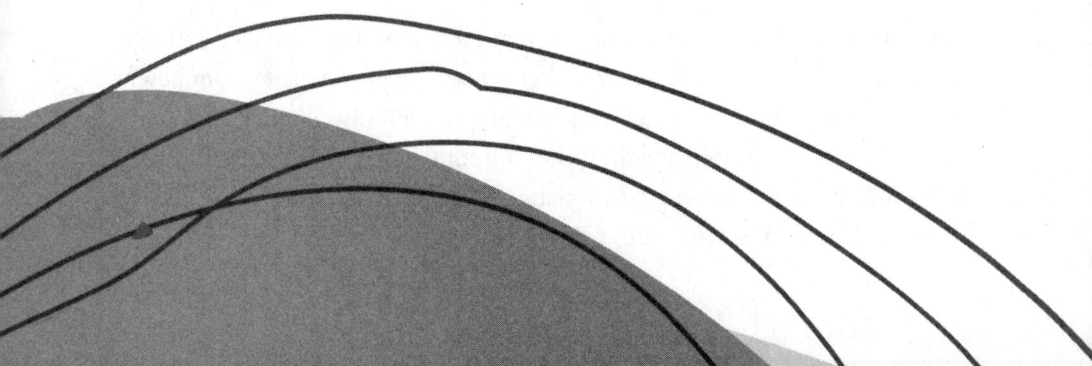

"What are you saying?*" cried George, as the doctor tried to explain what had happened. George's wife, Karen, had gone in for a very ordinary, quick procedure. They even had dinner plans! However, during the procedure a mistake had been made with the oxygen delivery, and Karen had been injured. As of right now, Karen wasn't waking up. George can't wrap his head around what the doctor is telling him. George is in shock.*

Karen does eventually wake up, but she's paralyzed on the right side of her body, which makes walking, writing, and speech very difficult. Karen gets fitted for a wheelchair, and the doctors don't offer any hope that she'll ever function as before. Karen and George can't really grasp the full breadth of life changes required; they're deep in the shock phase.

For Juan and Peter, it's different. Juan, a sous chef, and Peter, a pastry chef, met at a fancy restaurant where they both worked, and over the years, their entire relationship has been centered around travel and food. They both love to travel, but when in Rome they're not at the Sistine Chapel; they're at La Pergola, one of the world's fanciest restaurants. Everything they talk about, adventure around, and eat is gourmet.

But last year, Juan started to be debilitated by headaches and fatigue. Sometimes at work his vision went blurry and he almost couldn't stand long enough to finish his work. After getting checked out, his doctor tells Juan he has type 2 diabetes, but he refuses to believe it. After all, diabetes will wreck everything he cares about. And Peter doesn't even know *how to love on someone without making them a fancy dessert. What will they even talk about? What will they do for fun? Juan and Peter are simply lost in denial.*

However your chronic illness or chronic pain announced itself, you can likely relate to one of these two scenarios. Either your life completely changed in an instant or a day, or gradually you felt unwell and life slipped into an unrecognizable form. Either circumstance required enormous shifts and changes in your relationship that you may never have had to navigate before. For instance, George and Kathy have always struggled with finances, and now they must retrofit their entire house, never mind all the medical bills and legal issues that neither of them excel at. Juan and Peter have never really deepened their relationship beyond talk and activities surrounding food—they haven't had to! They have no idea what to talk about and do now.

The Lay of the Land

Every relationship has a rhythm, a pattern that has developed over time—some healthy and some unhealthy. You already have set ways that you communicate, express emotion and handle disagreements. When chronic illness arrives, it becomes an overlay on top of these already established rhythms. Don't expect to suddenly be able to communicate and handle this well if you have no established pattern for that. This new reality makes everything *more* complex, not less.

In this phase there's also a lag between entering the new reality and the couple's ability to handle their daily life within it. Whether the news is shocking or gradual, partners tend to still think they can operate as they always have. Only slowly does it dawn on them that this is no longer going to work. It's in this lag time that you experience that shock and denial; not ready yet to face what has happened, you're in the suspended void of not actually knowing *what* to feel, think, or do.

Not only that, but each individual experiencing this disorientation is also experiencing it together with the partner, as a unit. Denial might be operating in one of the partners, or the partners may be entering into denial together, making it very difficult to do anything differently. I don't mean that partners sit down and agree to be in denial together, but if there's something hard to face in life and your partner isn't addressing it, it's easy to just go along with the status quo. It's almost like an additional person has joined the relationship, and now everyone involved has to figure out how to navigate what has suddenly created a huge shift.

Communication and Emotions

Communication between partners and expressing emotions is especially difficult in this phase because partners generally don't even *know* what they're feeling! How can they express what they don't even know? Emotions are somewhat numbed, so there is sometimes just a sense of looking at one another with shaking heads and confused expressions, not knowing what on earth to say. Denial and shock serve a very important purpose—to protect you from getting totally overwhelmed by a change that's occurred. But it's often really hard to talk through these emotions, because by definition they're not grounding emotions, but *dissociative* emotions: You aren't really feeling anything, as opposed to feeling too much. Learning to communicate and feel your way through this stage takes some doing.

Sometimes in your pre-illness relationship, shared activity or busyness has been substituted for real communication. Now you're slowed down with inactivity or illness and you must learn to talk about things rather than practice escapism. Different coping mechanisms can come into play as well; some want to talk the issue into the ground, and others want to retreat into emotional avoidance.

In addition, the sick partner may feel like what is happening is happening solely to them and may be in denial that their partner is also experiencing something life-changing. They may feel like their partner can't possibly understand anything that they might be feeling, or that they can't talk to their partner because their partner won't get it. While this is technically true, both partners are experiencing a huge shift in their lives, and just because only one of them is ill does not mean they're the only person suffering.

Shared Activity

Whether you've suffered an extreme event such as Karen's on the operating table or a gradual onset like Juan's diabetes, your shared activity will likely be affected. Some people habitually numb their stronger emotions with a flurry of activity, but that may no longer be possible, depending on how the illness has affected the ability to move and get around.

Many couples have a pattern of shared activities, both around the house and recreationally. If one partner is now completely disabled, as Karen is, their shared activity will be completely curtailed. All of the chore type activities will now fall completely on George, and George also may feel like he can't or shouldn't engage in anything recreational. During the shock phase, however, shared activity is probably not even on anyone's radar. During shocking events, often family and friends jump in to help with chores and details, and recreational activity is far from anyone's mind.

In gradual cases of denial, like Juan's and Peter's, there may be an impulse to simply continue on as before and not talk about how shared activity will be impacted by the change that has occurred. For example, if Juan and Peter had a wine and cheese pairing at a winery coming up next weekend, it might not occur to them that they might need to moderate or change the activity because of this new development. Or denial may be operating solely in one person, while the other person doesn't know how to shift shared activity without the other person's buy-in.

Intimacy and Sex

During this phase intimacy may either increase or decrease, depending on whether the established pattern uses intimacy as a comfort activity. Some people may find touching and intimacy expresses all the things they are not yet able to express in words to their partner. Others may be so consumed with what has happened that sex and intimacy has taken a seat far back in the mind, and touching becomes the last thing they're interested in. Still others cannot engage in intimacy in the old ways because the injury or illness itself prevents it.

In shocking events, intimacy usually moves to the back burner. Because many partners consider intimacy *only* as sexual activity, there may be a lack of any touch at all—a shame, because touch is very healing. Partners will need to revert to an earlier way of thinking (think teenage years before you actually *had* intercourse) where all kinds of touch is exciting and interesting. And of course, initially, just comforting touch may be all the intimacy that's needed or required.

In cases of denial, sex and intimacy may continue much as before, but one partner may be exacerbating their symptoms—such as fatigue or pain—by engaging in the same level of intimate activity when it really should be modified. Sexual activity—like other comfort activities such as shopping, eating, gambling, and so on—can be used as a numbing or denial activity, and both partners should be alert for this. However, as I've said, denial serves a good purpose temporarily in terms of giving our mind a break from being overwhelmed. And if sexual activity is helpful and doesn't harm the sick partner, it may be okay to engage in more sexual activity in this phase to provide comfort and a distraction.

Friends, Family, and Gatekeeping

Another significant shift in this phase is communicating and getting support from others. If this is a gradual illness—unlike a sudden, urgent injury—perhaps it doesn't need to be communicated to family and friends yet. Either way, deciding what's shared and how it's shared is crucial. If the partners are experiencing this phase differently and not communicating well, this can become a real problem. One person might really need support from family and friends and need to talk a lot about what's happening, while the other person wants to keep the details private. Coming to some agreement about what is shared during this phase will set the stage for how and what to share in all of the coming phases.

Denial, in particular, is contagious in that, if you're denying the reality of an illness or injury, those around you are likely to join in your denial. As in the case of intimacy, partners may continue with all kinds of planned social activity, even though this level of activity may be damaging to their health in ways they refuse to see. The people around you will take your cues, and if you're in denial they also will minimize what you're dealing with and provide less of the support you may be wanting or needing.

Gatekeeping is the process through which information is filtered for dissemination. By gatekeeping, I mean the way in which partners decide what information should go out to the public—meaning friends, family, medical doctors, and so forth. If you're in denial, the medical community isn't going to be knocking at your door, asking you to address issues you don't want to address. Having a chronic illness requires a *lot* of advocating for yourself medically, and obviously if *you're* in denial, you won't be able to do that. Some partners may be wanting a lot of support and answers from the medical field; others, steeped in denial, may think they need no support whatsoever. It's important to decide what your roles will be if you attend appointments or talk to doctors together. Who will advocate? Who should speak, and what should they say?

Reflection Questions

1. Do you identify more with feelings of shock or feelings of denial? Do you resonate with the description I've provided for you?
2. Of the categories listed, what are your main concerns? Are you more upset by emotions, friends and family, gatekeeping?
3. How have you tried to cope with these concerns?

Coping with Shock and Denial

If you're in a phase of shock and denial, you aren't yet fully capable of really seeing what the future will hold, nor of solving the problems that will come. You may feel a disconnection with your own body, and feel unable to articulate anything you're feeling, to either yourself or your partner. That's why I've paired this section with the ACT skill of *being present*, because learning to just inhabit your own mind and body—in whatever stage you're in—will be important to what you're experiencing now, and to everything to come.

ACT Skill: Be Present Here and Now

Have you ever been driving somewhere and when you arrive, you really can't remember the drive? You wonder if lights were red or green, because you have no recollection of the process of driving yourself to your destination? Almost all of us have experienced this, with either driving or some other activity that we do so regularly we can drift off in our mind while we're doing it. This is clearly the opposite of being present.

Humans are generally not naturally skilled at staying present; our minds tend to drift off to either the past or the future, or just go on autopilot and zone out from what we're actually doing. This isn't *always* a bad thing; our minds sometimes *do* need a break from thinking and concentrating. But this zoning out, or disassociating, is particularly notable during the shock and denial phase of illness, when you're either consumed with how your past life looked or just unable to face whatever might be coming.

Being present is the practice of simply observing all of your experiences nonjudgmentally, whether internal or external. You're not concerned about what's happened in the past or may happen in the future, but just focused on what's happening right here, right now. Once, at a meditation retreat, the leader said "The present moment is *always* nonproblematic." There was a lot of argument on that one, and I still don't know if I can 100-percent agree, but you do have to admit that what is happening *right now* is usually not a problem. Usually what *has* happened, or what you fear *will* happen is the problem. Right now is usually a pretty okay place to be. But with illness or pain, sometimes you definitely do *not* like what is happening right now, so you revert to shock or denial. But as Byron Katie says (2002, p. 156), "when you argue with reality, you lose; but only 100 percent of the time!"

Learning to be present, in your body, with whatever that means right now, will be crucial to figuring out not only what you need to do next, but also what you can do as partners together. When you can feel what is going on within you and you're present for that, you're not in denial. And if you're in shock, learning how to be present with yourself can reground you in what is real instead of getting lost in a state of dissociation. When I used to teach meditation, the most common feedback I got was "I'm not good at meditation." And I would say "*No one* is good at meditation! That's why we call it a practice." Learning to be present is the same—it's an ongoing practice that you may not feel very good at, but if you keep practicing, you will definitely see the results.

ACT is famous for its metaphors that help us understand the concepts. For being present, we talk about how our minds are like a time machine. Your mind can travel back in time, and it's almost like you're actually there—that moment before you went into surgery, or the moment before the doctor said "It's diabetes." Or your mind can travel forward in time to that vacation you've got planned that you won't be able to take, or that meal you thought you were going to enjoy but now you know you won't. And what's the solution to the time machine? To "drop anchor."

Being present is like being in a boat in a storm, and you drop the anchor so you can just take stock of where you are and not drift, but find stability.

The main instruction for being present is simple: just "notice X." For example, notice the room you're in right now. What are the colors? What's the temperature? What kinds of textures can you feel? Is there a smell or a noise? Using your five senses, you can simply notice what *is* without making any changes whatsoever. This kind of noticing can keep you grounded in the moment as a starting point to come back into your body and the moment you're in.

Now let's see how staying present, using this tool, can help our example couples when they're in shock and denial:

George is sitting with Karen (who is still unconscious) in her hospital room when the doctor comes in to speak with him. The doctor gives George all kinds of overwhelming information, some of which he doesn't even understand. Family members are calling and visiting and wanting George to share this information, and it's all just too much. George's tendency is to just completely shut down; he turns on the hospital room TV and just zones out watching news. After all, there's always something going on in the news!

If George were going to try to be present now, he might try this: After the doctor spews all of his information, George might say "That was a lot of information; I'm going to take some time to digest it, and I might have more questions next time I see you." Then George walks to the window. He takes five deep breaths, breathing into his belly. He asks himself what is happening now—how does his body feel, what emotions he can identify, what does he see out the window? After doing this, he feels more grounded, and he sits down to try to write a list of things he heard the doctor say so he doesn't have to think about all of it at once.

Juan is more in denial than in shock, so he's more into the strategy of keeping busy. Juan is making plans with Peter, having lots of sex, inviting friends over, and taking on extra shifts at work. Juan is trying to prove to himself and others that he is fine, just fine. Nothing is wrong with him! He is conscious of headaches and fatigue, and he's expending lots of energy trying to pretend that he's not experiencing what he is actually experiencing.

If Juan were to practice being present, he would need to slow down, way down. It's not that Juan is completely debilitated like Karen, but he does need to make some serious changes in his life. He might not be completely ready to take everything in at this point, but he can start the process of change by being still and taking in what is happening.

Because Juan loves food, he begins by practicing mindfulness while he's preparing diabetic-friendly food. He knows he's going to need to eat differently, and there are actually some healthy recipes in his repertoire. So he practices being present while he's chopping vegetables. He notices the texture, the smells, the colors. He really concentrates on what his hands are doing, as if he has never done it before. This practice places Juan in a new relationship with food and also grounds him in the present moment, instead of avoiding any thought of change.

Reflection Questions

1. Looking back at your main concerns, how do you think learning to be present might help you with those?
2. Can you think of a time since this illness appeared that you had a present moment? Did it change the way you experienced things, or lead to better solutions?

Chapter Summary Points

- If the illness came on suddenly, as in the case of an accident, you're probably feeling shocked. If it came on gradually, you may be in denial, thinking things can soon go back to how they were.
- Communication is key here, because you're both either having a lot of feelings or trying to identify what you're feeling, so talking together about what those things are is crucial.
- Shared activity may have completely stopped—or continued as if nothing at all is wrong, if you're in denial. It's important to redefine what's possible in terms of shared activity.
- Intimacy may either increase or decrease, depending on whether this is a comfort activity for you—and you may feel differently about sex at this point, which is okay.
- It's important during this phase to define and ask for what kind of support you want to receive from your friends, family, and medical team.
- Learning the skill of being present in the moment is key here. It will help you come back into the truth of what is really happening and will help you shed the shock or denial of learning about this condition. The exercises in the following chapter will help you develop this skill.

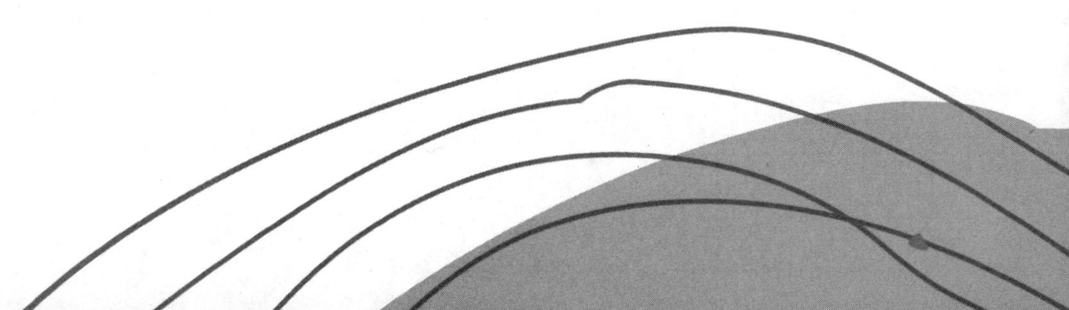

Moving On

I hope you can see how shock and denial play out for partners who are just learning about their chronic illnesses. Obviously, there are as many patterns as there are relationships, but I've tried to demonstrate some of the ways that partners can react. I also hope you can see how the practice of learning to be present can be helpful as you navigate this huge change in your lives. Now let's get into some specifics for how you each may be feeling and adjustments that you may need to make.

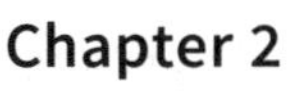

Chapter 2

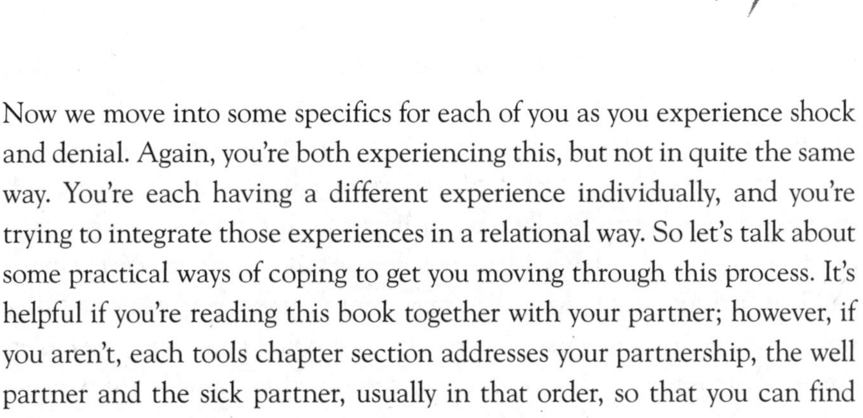

Tools for Shock and Denial

Now we move into some specifics for each of you as you experience shock and denial. Again, you're both experiencing this, but not in quite the same way. You're each having a different experience individually, and you're trying to integrate those experiences in a relational way. So let's talk about some practical ways of coping to get you moving through this process. It's helpful if you're reading this book together with your partner; however, if you aren't, each tools chapter section addresses your partnership, the well partner and the sick partner, usually in that order, so that you can find information specific to what you're coping with.

How You May Be Feeling

A bomb has just gone off in your lives. Whatever your patterns have been in the past, this will magnify them, so try to be gentle with each other. It's not too late to learn healthier ways of relating, even if your interactions haven't been so healthy.

Well Partner

Whether an accident has occurred or your partner has revealed a diagnosis, your life as the well partner has changed without your having a choice in the matter. If you're feeling shock, you may feel like your head is spinning; if you're in denial, you may feel resistance to having to make any changes in your life. Every single person is different; I can't know your circumstances or predict how you're feeling.

Sick Partner

Your life just changed in ways you never predicted. Obviously, this portion of the chapter describes your feelings once you're aware that you're not well. If that change is catastrophic, as Karen's was, there's no possible way to deny what has happened, but you will be in shock. You had a full calendar, just as we all do, and now everything has to be shifted. You may be the type to retreat in shock and not want to talk to anyone or do anything, or you may be the type who pulls in all the support you can find.

If you've experienced a long slide of symptoms or have recently gotten a chronic illness diagnosis like Juan did, you might be feeling more denial. It might be a relief to finally have a diagnosis, but now it puts you in a category—you have a label. Many people don't like that and don't want to be identified in such a group. You may want to prove you're "not all that sick" or otherwise resist making changes that could make your life easier. Again, there is no cookie-cutter way to describe this phase, so think of my descriptions and suggestions as just that—suggestions.

Communication and Emotions

Try to remember now that *one* of you is sick, but *both* of you are suffering myriad losses in your lives. During the phase of shock and denial, you don't have to make sense of everything you're feeling, but do set aside some regular times to sit together so you can talk about anything you might be feeling. We all deal with things in different ways; it's unlikely that you're dealing with this in the same way. Learn active listening during this phase; it will help you throughout the entire process. Active listening simply means listening with the intent not to respond, but to completely understand.

You will both be feeling an array of emotions underneath the numbness that comes with shock or denial. You might not realize at first how complex the emotions are—dismayed, startled, confused, helpless, scared, worried, overwhelmed—I could go on. It's helpful to move out of numbness and get clear on what you're feeling, because then you can communicate from that space rather than a numb place. This will make your communication smoother. Take a look at the feelings chart at the end of this section. See if you can identify any emotions you might be feeling right now.

Well Partner

When communicating with your partner, see if speaking from these emotions helps you clarify what you're trying to say. For example, if you say "I'm worried about how we will adjust to this new reality, but I'm confident we can figure it out," that's likely to get a productive response from your partner and generate good conversations. Become aware if you're an internal processor (emotional withdrawal) or an external processor (need to talk about things), so that you can evaluate whether you need to express more of your emotions or find new ways of externalizing your feelings.

Sick Partner

As a newly diagnosed person, your emotions might be blunted, or you might be feeling incredible shifts of all kinds of emotions, leaving you overwhelmed. This is *your* illness, but it likely affects everyone around you as well. It's good to try to get a handle on your emotions so you can communicate what you're feeling and the changes that are going on. You might set aside particular times to communicate about it, especially if you're struggling with denial. This allows you to "live normally" for some periods of the day, but have specific time periods when you talk with your partner about how you're feeling and the changes that need to be made.

Be gentle with yourselves. This is probably something you've never experienced before, and no emotion is off limits. Even if you feel a little frozen, just let it be. This time period is about putting one foot in front of the other until you start to feel motivation to move forward.

EXERCISE: Identifying Feelings

Look at the emotions chart below. The core emotions are boldface; those below them are more nuanced versions. See if you can identify a feeling you're having or have had recently. Close your eyes for a few moments and try to see where you feel that in your body. What does it feel like? Is it static, or moving around? Take some deep breaths and try to visualize that feeling moving through you like water. We want you to move from numbness, shock, and denial to actually feeling and naming your emotions, so try to do this exercise a couple of times each day.

Sad	**Angry**	**Fearful**
Depressed	Frustrated	Anxious
Powerless	Annoyed	Excluded
Disappointed	Numb	Overwhelmed
Abandoned	Resentful	Frightened
Despair	Betrayed	Helpless

EXERCISE: Daily Communication

Set aside fifteen minutes a day where you'll try to communicate with each other how you're feeling. Remember that you may feel differently from each other, and that's okay. It might be helpful to have a timer so this time does not become overwhelming. Take turns talking for five minutes each about whatever is on your mind; the listening partner simply listens without any judgment of what their partner is saying. This is a practice of being present, not problem solving. If either partner talks about something that needs to be handled or solved, write it down in a notebook to be taken care of later.

Shared Activity

Shared activity takes a hit during this stage, but the hope is to maintain your connection so that when you want to pick things back up later, there's still a desire to spend time with your partner. During this period, try to spend some time together doing sedentary things like watching shows you like or that can make you laugh or otherwise distract you from the seriousness of your lives. Try to think of how you spend this time not as avoidance of your feelings, but as a way to connect with each other in a shared activity that you can talk or laugh about together later.

Well Partner

Right now, your main activity is likely a focus on treatments and healing modalities that your partner needs. Getting the right medical help really can be a full-time job, and it's important to remember that you need to take breaks and take care of yourself in order to make it through this process in a healthy way. If you and your partner have always done certain activities together, like going to the gym, you may have to do those things alone for a while—maybe for a long while. If you need to start modifying plans—for example, if your partner is regularly fatigued—try making plans to meet up with a friend on your own for now. You'll need to learn a new level of independence now, and there's no time like the present to begin. Remember that your partner may have complicated feelings around your making plans without them; continue to communicate and be considerate of those feelings. For example, you might say "You know I'd rather play pickleball with you than with anyone else, but I want you to take care of yourself right now, and my playing with Frank doesn't mean that I'm leaving you behind. We'll find ways to do things together as we adapt."

Sick Partner

As the sick partner, you most likely have an established pattern of shared activities with your partner. You may not be able to participate in any of these activities right now, or you may need to adjust them. There are likely some that you should curtail right now, and it's good to be clear about this with your partner. Try to think of some ways you two *could* share some activities that feel good for you. For example, Juan and Peter have always cooked luscious meals together, and Juan feels like he can't do that after his diabetes diagnosis. But he suggests that maybe he and Peter could watch some cooking shows they've been meaning to watch. This honors their connection without exhausting Juan or creating food he can't eat.

It's also okay if you don't feel like doing any activity with your partner for a short period. In this case, try to communicate that you do like doing things together and that you'll figure out together a way to get back there someday. Your partner will appreciate hearing you say something like "I love doing things together with you. I can't do that now, but it's a major goal of mine to figure out how to spend time together as we go forward." If you yourself are not capable of activity right now, it's a loving gift to encourage your partner to go engage in some activity on their own, though it may be hard to watch.

EXERCISE: Increasing Self-Care

Identify some self-care activities that are possible for you during this process. It's crucially important to have ways to take care of yourself as you're adjusting to this new life. Things that involve going outside, being with people, and moving your body, if possible, can be particularly healing. These can be small pockets of time; no need to commit to major chunks of time.

Intimacy and Sex

Many people equate intimacy and sex. However, when one person becomes ill, you may have to find new definitions of intimacy that are pleasing to you both. During the first phase of shock and denial, you may not want to have sex at all. This is fine. However, touch is enormously healing for humans, and it'll help you maintain a physical connection—even if all you can do is sit closer on the couch watching TV.

Well Partner

You may still be well, but you've been sick before; we all have. So you can understand how, when you're not feeling well, sex is really not on your mind. In fact, sex may actually be impossible, at least for a while, as in Karen's case. But remember that intimacy is much more than sex. Ask your partner if gentle touch would feel good for them, or what kind of sensual touch might be comforting. Perhaps just hugs work for now. If you can, identify what your own needs are and see if there are some that your partner could meet, even though they are sick. For example, it might feel nice just to lie together skin to skin without anything else happening.

Know that intimacy is going to change, and for now, try to practice patience as you adapt to your new lifestyle. If you've been in denial about a health problem, your sexual activity may not be changed by the diagnosis. But if you're not the one in denial, pay attention to how sexual activity affects your partner, in terms of things like pain and fatigue. You might be able to suggest some new ideas that accommodate your partner better, such as slowing down, reducing frequency, and highlighting lower-energy activities like snuggling. It can be very healing for your partner to hear you say something like "It's okay with me if we can't do [fill in] as often right now. I understand."

Sick Partner

Sex and intimacy might be the *last* thing on your mind while experiencing shock—it might not even be possible, depending on your illness. But again, remember that over time you and your partner will have to readjust, and it can be helpful to reassure your partner that you'll be up for that in the future, even if you can't imagine it now.

On the other hand, if you're experiencing some kind of denial, you may not want to change anything about how you interact, *or* you might even be feeling increased desire because touch feels reassuring to you. Since most chronic illnesses involve some kind of fatigue and pain, just be careful to not overdo it. Intimacy involves all kinds of sensual touch; perhaps you can add some pleasures that involve gentle touch for comfort and relief. It can be comforting to both partners if you say what you need in advance, like "I don't have the energy for sex right now, but could we just hold each other skin to skin without any pressure?"

EXERCISE: Mindful Touch

Try a practice of mindful touch. Again, this is about being present in the moment and experiencing the healing connection of touch. You can simply lie together, possibly skin to skin, without talking or otherwise touching. Almost all sick partners can do this. There is no active touch here, or anything leading to further intimacy.

Another idea is for the well partner to lie back against a couch or bed headboard, and the sick partner lies back against their partner's chest, facing the same direction. The well partner can wrap their arms around their partner for stability. This can be clothed or unclothed. No need to talk or otherwise move in any way. Just lie silently and feel each other's breathing, possibly syncing your breathing rhythm patterns.

Friends, Family, and Gatekeeping

You'll have to decide how much contact you want with friends and family, and what type. In this first phase, it's fine if you don't want to see them at all. It can be complicated to explain what is happening, and you may not feel like small talk. Or together you may decide on a few people who would be helpful to connect with; if so, do that and explain exactly what would be helpful to you both.

Decide now what information will be shared by each of you, and how. For example, it can be a huge betrayal for the well partner to post on Facebook if the sick partner wants to be more private about what's happening. This early stage of your journey will set the tone for all of the information sharing throughout this process, so have an open discussion about it now.

Well Partner

In cases like Juan's and Peter's, when the illness onset is or has been gradual, you may not have communicated anything yet to your friends and family. But in cases like George's and Karen's, everyone may know what's going on. Either way, others may share your shock and denial. It's hard to be in your own shock and try to figure out how to manage other people's. As the well partner, it might be good to designate one person to let everyone else know and later to update. Also, talk to your partner now about what they want shared, and what—if anything—is off limits. This will change as the process unfolds, but for now you need some ground rules.

You may be in charge at this point of working with the doctors on decision making, as George had to be after Kathy's incident. If so, include your partner if possible in those discussions. If this is a gradual-onset illness, figure out whether your partner wants you to come to doctors' visits, and if so, whether you should talk, take notes, or just listen.

Sick Partner

Depending on your personality (and other factors), friends and family might be completely overwhelming you, or you may want more of their attention than they can give. Few of us are very good at dealing with crises like this, and be prepared: People may say all manner of ridiculous things. Try not to be too offended; we have no training in what to say in these circumstances, so it's best to receive these statements in the spirit in which they're offered. Many people will try to offer "get well soon" type wishes, not understanding the nature of chronic illnesses. You don't need to correct and educate at this point. Find your own balance; that will help you develop a balance with others.

Sharing information at this stage is fraught with difficulty; again, try designating one person to relay information to your circle of support. Also, you're now sick and interacting with many medical professionals, and you need to decide if you'd like your partner to be part of those conversations, if that's an option. You also need to figure out your partner's role in these conversations. Do you want them to ask questions and possibly speak for you, or to remain silent and just take notes? If you don't really know what you want, don't worry: You'll know what you *don't* want if it happens; and if it does, be gentle with your partner and just explain that this doesn't work for you and needs to change. When this happens, calm yourself down with box breathing (see instructions in a following exercise); then you'll be able to have a more productive discussion.

EXERCISE: Grounding in the Moment

There are many ways to ground yourself in the present moment. It's too early to know everything about what you're feeling and your particular situation. Being right here, right now is useful. One way is to use all the senses available to you. Look around where you are right now. Name something you can see. Name something you can hear. Name something you can smell, or touch, or taste. Take a moment to really notice each sensation, almost as if you've never experienced it before. Appreciate how you can still experience pleasure through your senses, even if other parts of your body don't work as you wish.

The main thing at this stage is to be gentle. Be gentle with yourself, with your partner, with your friends and family. This is a new experience for everyone; no one knows yet what is helpful or not, and you're all struggling with shock and denial and trying to sort out your feelings.

EXERCISE: Box Breathing

One thing that's always happening in the moment is your breath. (Some chronic illnesses that affect respiration, such as COPD, may require adapting this exercise.) If it's safe for you, try doing a "box breath." Inhale for a count of four (or whatever number works for you); hold at the top of the inhale for four; exhale for four counts; hold at the bottom of the exhale for four. That's one round. Doing five of those will help ground you in the moment. It's hard to think about anything else while you're counting, and for these few moments you're solidly in the moment. If you do have COPD or another respiratory disease, try just observing your breath. Notice how your belly rises and falls, or the feeling of air going in and out of your nostrils. Try choosing a place in your body where you notice the breath, and just observe the inhales and exhales for a few minutes, as if you've never noticed this before. If your mind wanders, that's okay. Just notice that too, and come back to your breathing.

Moving On

I hope you've found some ways to navigate through shock and denial. This phase might be brief or longer lasting. Remember, you may revisit this phase as new symptoms or diagnoses arise, or at different points in your life. This is normal, and if that occurs, I invite you to reread this chapter.

The next likely phase is anger, as your feelings become more recognizable. Anger is a very tough emotion for many, but it's possible to find your way through it with grace. Let's talk about how!

Chapter 3

Anger Phase

What You Will Learn in This Chapter:

- There's *so* much to be angry about, but partners are often angry about different things.
- It's helpful to look at anger as a signal of something that needs to be changed.
- Suppressing anger does not help; learning to communicate what you're angry about is very helpful for partners.
- The tool of defusion, "unhooking" from your thoughts, is a good way to get a handle on anger.
- Not all thoughts are true, even though they may be valid.
- Getting some distance and perspective on your feelings of anger can help you communicate them to your partner.

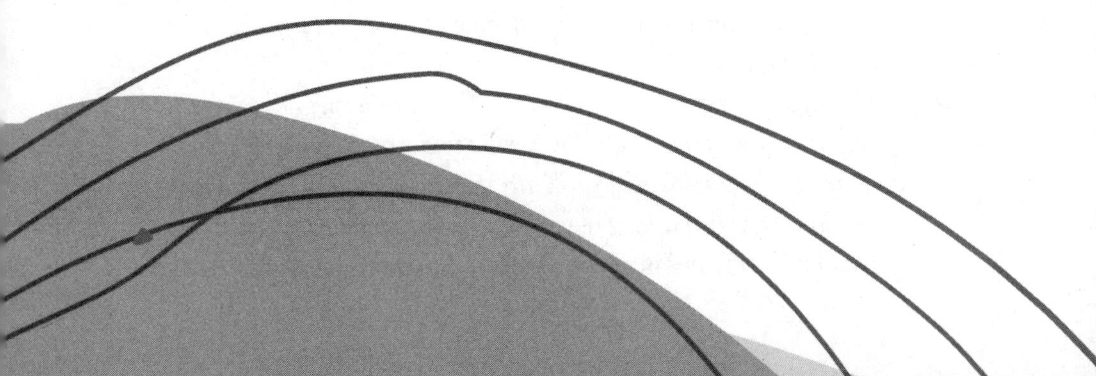

Sam is raging. Once again, Juliette says she can't attend the party they're having at his workplace. He's been looking forward to it for so long, and she knows this. But Juliette is having her period, and as usual, she's writhing in pain. Or so she says; Sam isn't so sure he really believes it anymore. Juliette told Sam that she's been diagnosed with endometriosis, but Sam has lived his life by the philosophy of just "pushing through"—why can't she just do that? He feels like he can't talk with her about how this affects him. He had the evening all planned in his mind, concluding with some fantastic sex, but that's not happening now. Sam wonders if it will ever really happen.

Juliette is pretty mad too. Obviously, she realizes that it's tough for Sam to understand her medical issues when he doesn't deal with them. But anyone can understand severe pain, can't they? Sam doesn't seem to make any effort. It's all about how this affects him, *and when Juliette tries to explain her pain, her fears, her despair, she gets dismissed. Not that she's not used to dismissal; after all, it took her years for the doctors to listen to her, even though there are over six million people diagnosed with endometriosis in the United States (Dusenbery 2018, p. 216). But shouldn't you be able to count on compassion from your partner?*

Mason and Jill have different issues. At thirty years old, Mason has been diagnosed with Leber's optic neuropathy, a hereditary disease that means he'll likely go blind in the next ten years or so. Jill is endlessly hopeful that they'll come up with a solution, which feels super dismissive to Mason and enrages him. But then when she meets him in his discouragement, that makes him mad too. He's mad when she tries to be helpful, and mad when she doesn't. He's mad about pretty much everything. He knows she is trying to help, but he can't even figure out what kind of help he wants, *so he's left with just a boatload of anger.*

Jill is a little angry as well. She feels like Mason isn't advocating for himself very well medically. She's gone to a few appointments with him, and he doesn't really ask any questions or follow up on any information. She tried asking questions and researching, but she gets her head bitten off, and then she's *mad. Who's going to ask the questions, then? It's so frustrating to try to be helpful, switch gears when that's not helpful, and then get yelled at again. Nothing she does seems to be working, and now her anger is just targeted at Mason. What's his problem, anyway?*

If you've been diagnosed with any kind of chronic illness, anger is probably a stage that you recognize. There is so *much* to be angry about, after all. From the moment of symptom onset, each partner is on a very different journey, so anger can erupt as one partner doesn't understand the other's experience. Anger is very uncomfortable for many people, so it's crucial that you get some tools for dealing with it in the context of chronic illness.

The Lay of the Land

Most of us think one thing about anger: It's bad, bad, bad. But it's *not* always bad. Anger is a vital emotion. If you never get angry, either you don't have any boundaries or you don't notice or care when people run roughshod over your boundaries. Anger is very motivating—it pushes us to do something different. In the case of chronic illness, anger can be what helps you to stand up for yourself and advocate for yourself, both of which you sorely need. And as Sarah Ramey says in her wonderful memoir, *The Lady's Handbook for Her Mysterious Illness*, "when anger finally surfaces, the patient is about to have a breakthrough" (2020, p. 86). So don't discount anger or feel like the only strategy is to get rid of it. You need anger, but you also need it to be healthy and expressed in healthy ways. And especially in a partnership, you need to manage anger so that you can get the support that you need from one another.

Communication and Emotions

I often tell my clients that trying to suppress emotion is like holding a beach ball underwater. You can do it for a while, but if a big enough wave comes along, it's going to pop right out! Most of us do try to suppress anger, because we've been told it's a bad feeling to have and express. When chronic illness strikes, people may fear expressing their anger because they feel like it's a contemptible thing to feel, but anger is a very *common* response to chronic illness, for so many reasons. People also may express anger inappropriately, because it seems easier to express than the hopelessness or sadness they may be feeling. The bottom line is that not talking productively about your feelings—even anger—is a disservice to everyone.

Further, many of the things you may be angry about—like fate or the medical community—aren't things that you can target with your anger, so your anger just gets turned on or "leaked" out onto the other. Or sometimes you get a little self-centered and feel like other people don't have it nearly as bad as you do, and you get impatient with what you see as their insignificant complaints. This especially happens with sick partners when they don't understand or see that their well partner also has valid struggles. In these ways, your anger is being directed toward people who don't deserve it, but it's a way to disperse the anger, even if it isn't solving the problem.

The main thing to understand is that anger is a *normal* and common response. It's important to find ways to communicate with each other about your anger, or about what creates angry feelings for you as you navigate this new landscape. Understanding that anger is normal makes it much easier to talk about it and try to figure out ways to interact that don't increase anger (see chapter 4 for some specific exercises).

Shared Activity

In this phase, the main issue with shared activity is that partners get angry because things have shifted. The well partner may be upset because activities the couple has habitually done together cannot continue as before. This is especially problematic if the well partner doesn't believe the sick partner or doesn't understand the severity of their symptoms. If you got together in the first place solely or largely based on a shared interest, and that interest is now curtailed, that can cause anger for both partners because they can't engage in the same activities, and for the sick partner because they're being pressured to do things they feel they can't do.

Sometimes the well partner *is* very respectful or deferential to the sick partner when it comes to activity, but forgets to be deferential in other areas. For example, a friend of mine described how her husband will tell her "be careful, be careful" while she is going down steps, but then leaves all the bathroom cleaning for her to do. All shared activity must be renegotiated, not just the fun stuff. You both can alleviate a lot of unnecessary conflict by sitting down to intentionally renegotiate basic life tasks.

Intimacy and Sex

There are some specific chronic illnesses that particularly affect sex—like Juliette's endometriosis, vulvodynia, and other reproductive conditions. But almost *all* chronic illnesses involve some kind of fatigue. So even if it's not a specific reproductive issue, intimacy can be impacted. Again, as with any shared activity, both partners may be angry that sex and intimacy cannot continue as before, and the sick partner may be angry that they're being pressured or asked to do things that they don't feel well enough to do.

Understand that anger is pretty normal here. Sex is already difficult to talk about for many partners, absent any external issues. For many partners, anger on this topic may already be brewing prior to the injury or illness. Well partners may pressure for more sex, *or* they may avoid the topic altogether in an attempt to not appear selfish; neither approach is sustainable. The sick partner's body has been "rezoned" as a medical site, so it's understandable that sex takes a backseat.

If you take the approach that anger brewing here as pretty normal, it might become easier to talk about it. Try to be gentle with each other and understand that if you're in a committed monogamous relationship, this need cannot be met anywhere else. So you'll need to discuss it over time—including *all* of the feelings it engenders—and come up with new solutions. If you're in a nonmonogamous relationship, you may have to revisit the terms of your previous agreements to accommodate the unwell partner(s).

If you're the sick partner, even just saying "I still want you and I understand how important sex is to both of us. I'm committed to finding ways of continuing our sexual connection, even if it's hard" can make a tremendous difference. Or if you're the well partner, you can say, without pressure or judgment, "I'm here to totally support you in this illness experience, and I'm not here to pressure you in ways that don't work for you. But over the long haul, I do want us to find ways to stay physically connected."

Friends, Family, and Gatekeeping

Both of you are trying to manage and adapt to this new phase in your life, but so is everyone who loves you. So anger can arise with friends and family, too. It's hard enough to manage your own thoughts and feelings without having to manage everyone around you. Depending on the varying ability of your friends and family to manage their own angst, you may be asked to comfort others when you're the one needing comfort. Clearly that's not your job, but you can feel pressure and overwhelm nonetheless—leading to anger.

In addition, many chronic illnesses are invisible; that is, you can't tell by observing that someone isn't feeling well. Think about how Juliette likely presents herself to the world: People probably see her as "normal." Juliette isn't going to go around telling everyone she has cramps or is bleeding profusely. No one will see that from the outside. So there's often a huge disconnect between how the sick partner feels inside and how others view them, prompting the common "But you don't *look* sick!" It's easy to get angry about not being supported. Understand that educating those around you is going to take some time and doesn't happen overnight. As Sarah Ramey says, "The level of invalidation is truly omnidirectional, it's unusual, and it *includes* your inner circle and what would normally be your support system" (2020, p. 307).

As we discussed in the previous chapter, gatekeeping governs how partners distribute information to the outside world. Anger comes up here because it takes time to learn how best to speak about what has happened, who should speak about it, to whom, and what they should say. The sick partner often has some competing interests; they want people to both stay out of their business *and* help them, to both not smother them *and* show them they care. The well partner is often doing the best they can to garner support from the outside world but is likely to make a few missteps while they try to figure it all out.

The sick partner will need to work on defining their own boundaries, and often they don't know that something is a boundary until someone has not honored that boundary, triggering anger. This anger is your friend, alerting you to something that isn't helpful. Try to see this as a very informative response, helping you to figure out over time what works for you and what doesn't. And if you're the well partner, try to take your partner's anger in stride; they're figuring all of this out, just as you are.

Let's turn for a moment to medical gaslighting. This isn't directly related to gatekeeping, although the well partner may need to take a role in this area to protect the sick partner. It's common for the partners (both individually and as a team) to feel anger toward the medical community. I wish I could say this is rare. In her 2018 book, *Doing Harm*, Maya Dusenbery talks at length about this issue. She explains that people with chronic illness are so often referred to mental health professionals—with a "diagnosis" that the patient must be just anxious or worried—that mental health professionals are often the first in the medical community to properly diagnose their diseases. There's a certain kind of rage reserved for being told that you don't experience what you experience, or that you can't possibly be feeling what you're feeling. Again, this anger is healthy, because the way we're often treated by doctors is so out of line.

Reflection Questions

1. How do you feel about anger? Were you allowed to be angry growing up? Has other people's anger ever harmed you?
2. What are you most angry about since the diagnosis of chronic illness?
3. How has your anger affected the way you interact with your partner?

Coping with Anger

The answer to anger isn't to shove it away or repress it. This rarely, if ever, works. But you also know that anger can be destructive, and destroying your relationships—especially with your partner—isn't the way to go either. So what can you do with your anger? Once again, ACT has some answers for us, in the form of cognitive defusion.

ACT Skill: Cognitive Defusion

Cognitive *what?* Don't let the confusing name bother you. As you know, we humans can get "hooked" by our thoughts, just like a fish on a line. We have a thought, and just automatically believe it's true, and then that leads us to all kinds of other thoughts and feelings that may or may not be helpful. Anger, in particular, is easy to get hooked into believing because it's such a physical experience that it seems like it *has* to be real or true.

But thoughts, however painful and intense, are not necessarily true. When you're in a fight or conflict, your angry thought—*You're so selfish!*—may feel very real and upsetting, but it's not necessarily true, or true all the time. It's simply a thought and a feeling. Now, I'm not invalidating strong thoughts and feelings; again, anger serves a valuable purpose and can give you some good information that you might need to pay attention to. Your thoughts and feelings of anger are absolutely *valid*, but that doesn't necessarily mean they are *true*. There's a big difference between the two.

So while respecting the feeling and thoughts of anger, also realize that defusion helps you create just a little distance from these thoughts and feelings; it helps you take a step back. These are just thoughts—normal thoughts—and may even have some truth. But to be effective and successful in your relationship, you must learn to get a little distance from your thoughts, so instead of just reacting to them, you can decide what to do about them.

For example, let's say you're drowning in an ocean. You see your suitcase floating nearby, filled with all the precious items you brought with you on your journey. You also see a life preserver. Both are valid things for you to grab onto, but only one of them is going to save you. Not that your suitcase isn't important; it is! There are many important things in there. But that isn't what you need to grab onto right now.

Your thoughts and feelings—especially anger—have a lot of value and contain important information. But they also may not be what you need right now, or what will work for you in a given situation. And to decide that, you'll need to be able to step back and assess the situation.

Well, great, you may say, *but how do I do that?* First, it can be helpful to think of your mind as an entity separate from you. In the same way that you can observe what is happening around you (a car just drove by, it was fast and red), you can also observe what your mind is doing. If you don't make this disconnection, you run the risk of just accepting and believing everything your mind tells you. If you think *I'm worthless*, then you believe that you're worthless. But if you see your mind as a thought-generating machine, you can be interested in the fact that your mind is *telling* you that you're worthless, then step back and assess whether that thought is useful or true.

Second, there are several techniques you can use to generate this kind of distance from your angry thoughts and feelings. I'll give you some specific exercises in the next chapter. But for now, I'll briefly explain a few techniques that might be helpful.

Write Thoughts Down

I know, it sounds ridiculously simple, but most of us do not have a really good running awareness of what our thoughts are doing. Writing your thoughts down automatically creates distance, because they're now just words on a paper, and it's easier to assess whether they're true or helpful. If you want to become more aware of your thoughts, put an alarm on your phone four or five times a day, and when the alarm goes off, just write down whatever you're thinking.

Thoughts as Stories

Your mind is a storytelling machine, and if you consider that thoughts you may have are simply stories, then you can get a little distance to assess whether this is just a fantastical story, or there's some truth to it. So if you're thinking about your partner *He's never going to get well, because he's so passive!* you can just say to yourself *Oh, there's the "he's never going to get well" story.* As we all know, some stories are true and some are fiction; some are useful and some are not. Seeing your thoughts as stories can help you make this assessment.

"I'm Having the Thought That"

Similarly, you can use this technique to find some distance. If you say to yourself *I'm always sick*, then "you" and "sick" are one and the same, completely fused together. But if you say *I notice that I'm having the thought that I'm always sick*, then there's "you," and there's the thought, but you're not necessarily connected. From that place, you can either discard that thought or change it to something more useful, like *I'm feeling sick right now, but I don't always*, or *Since I'm feeling sick today, I will go back to sleep* and so forth.

Silly Songs or Voices

Many people have great success taking a troublesome thought and either singing it to a catchy tune or saying it out loud in a silly voice. This isn't to disrespect the thought or feeling, but to remove a little of its gravity and seriousness. If you can be silly or laugh at a thought, then it's easier to disconnect from it and therefore be able to take a step back and assess whether it's true or helpful.

Leaves, Clouds, Birds

Many images that people use for their thoughts help give a little bit of distance. You can think of your thoughts like leaves on a river, and you're the river. The leaves are not attached to the river; they just float on by without becoming a part of the river. Similarly, you can think of your thoughts like clouds in the sky, drifting along—some dark, some puffy—but either way, coming and going without damaging the sky. Birds flying in the sky, cars going by on the freeway—lots of possibilities. Whatever image appeals to you is a good way to simply observe that your thoughts are coming and going without becoming attached to them.

Reflection Questions

1. Does the skill of cognitive defusion seem helpful to gain perspective on your anger?
2. Have you ever been able to "unhook" from an angry thought? Did that change the way you behaved next?

Chapter Summary Points

- Anger is a completely normal and appropriate emotion to have when chronic illness strikes.
- Often partners are angry at the medical system, other people, and the illness itself—but then take this anger out on each other in inappropriate ways.
- Trying to suppress your anger won't make the anger go away.
- Learning to see anger as a positive signal that lets you know something is amiss is helpful.
- It's very important to learn to talk with your partner calmly about what causes anger for them so you can collaborate on solutions.
- Cognitive defusion is the ACT tool for anger; this means to stop believing everything you think, and instead get a little distance and perspective on those thoughts.
- It's helpful to see our minds as storytellers and our thoughts as stories.

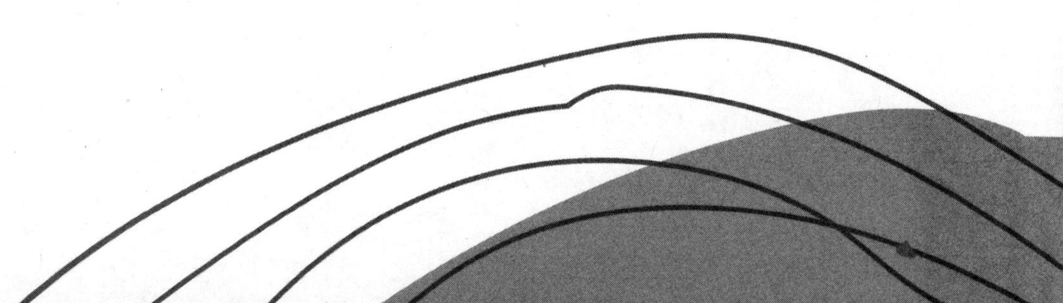

Moving On

I hope I've made my points: Angry feelings and thoughts can be useful and give you good information, but those thoughts need not control your behavior. And anger is entirely normal in adjusting to the arrival of a chronic illness in your relationship. The more you can view this as a normal way of processing information, the better you can communicate about and use that information. One way is to work on techniques of cognitive defusion so that angry feelings and thoughts don't overwhelm you and control your actions in a damaging way. Now let's talk about some specific ways that you can work with anger, both individually and as a partnership.

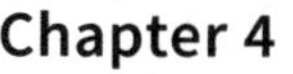

Chapter 4

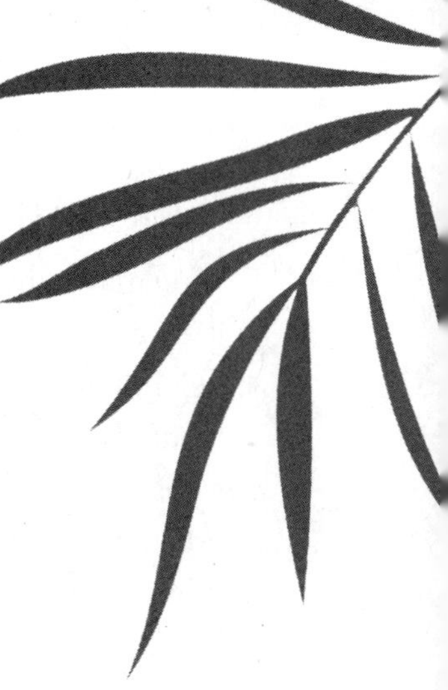

Tools for the Anger Phase

As you add more concrete tools, remember that it's *normal* and healthy to feel anger as you're getting used to life with a chronic illness. You're not trying to eliminate anger in this process, but you'll try to cope with these feelings and learn to interact with one another supportively as you're experiencing it.

How You May Be Feeling

Your lives have been upended in ways that you didn't anticipate, and there are more things to be angry about than you know how to handle. To top it off, you're probably angry about different things, which makes it hard to work together. Let's talk about some of the minefields and how to navigate them.

Well Partner

You and your body are still operating at the same functionality as before your partner got sick. Clearly their life has changed, but what are you supposed to do with the fact that you haven't changed at all, yet your life is upside down? This sense of unfairness and change can lead to a lot of anger on your end, and you need to learn how to deal with it.

Sick Partner

You may normally be comfortable with anger, or suppress it, or respond to it in destructive ways. Whatever your pattern has been before with occasional anger, it's likely pronounced now, because you're probably angry *all the time.* Something's happened to you that you didn't cause, that will change your life in myriad ways and will never fully be healed or cured. How on earth could you *not* be angry? But if you didn't do any work on anger prior to your illness, you're going to need to work on it now.

Communication and Emotions

Anger is a difficult emotion and hard to talk about in the best of times. You need a way to talk to one another about the anger you're both feeling and the judgments you may be making. The well partner may think the sick partner shouldn't be as angry, because all of the practical burdens are falling on them. The sick partner may think the well partner has no right to be angry, because after all, they are still well. It'll help from the get-go if you both acknowledge that there's plenty to be angry about on both sides, and agree not to judge one another for angry feelings. Setting aside some specific time to talk about what's making you angry can be quite helpful. It's important to put a real container around these conversations, so that the anger doesn't "leak" out over your whole existence. If you agree to twenty minutes, set a timer. Each of you can talk for ten minutes about all of the things that are making you feel angry. Problem solving can come later; try to just listen and empathize with your partner's experience.

Well Partner

Most of us are uncomfortable with anger. You might deal with it in one of two ways—either you hold all of that anger in and pretend everything is going along fine, or you burst forth in anger in destructive or uncomfortable ways. You probably realize that neither response feels very good or productive. Try to allow anger to simply exist without needing to do anything about it. For some, this is a life-changing practice—to realize that feeling something does not necessarily mean something needs to be done about it.

Sick Partner

Again, the emotion of anger is *normal.* It totally makes sense that you're angry, and you've every right to be. How to deal with and talk about this is another story. It may be helpful to keep a running list of all of the things that you're angry about, because there will be a lot! You may communicate your anger to others without actually saying that you're angry, so learning to be clearer can be useful. Most people around you will understand that you feel angry. So start a practice of saying "I'm feeling angry about…" Also, it can be useful to prep the person you're talking to that you'll be talking about anger, and to let them know what you need from the conversation; for example, "I'd like to talk to you about some things that I'm feeling angry about, and I actually don't need anything from you but to just sit and listen to what I have to say," or "I'd like to talk to you about some things I'm feeling angry about, and when I'm finished, I'd like your help trying to figure out some solutions." Doing this will help the other person (who is probably also uncomfortable with anger) to give you what you need.

EXERCISE: Communicate about Anger

Set aside some time to talk about things that anger each of you. Set a specific time and divide the time so you both have time to talk (you can start brief, like twenty minutes total, so you each get ten minutes to talk). Before you begin, remind each other that anger is a normal emotion and it's healthy to talk about it. And also that you may not be in the solution phase yet, and that it's okay to just listen. If you're the listener, try to "unhook" from the content of the conversation. In other words, listen carefully to what your partner is saying, but think about the room you're in as a river, and each thing your partner is saying is just a leaf floating by. Or a freeway, and each thought is just a car driving by. Allow it to be present and then float past. Not in a dismissive way, just in a nonattached way.

EXERCISE: Notice Your Anger

Learning to unhook from your anger means separating out the *feeling* of anger from the *behavior* of anger. Check in with yourself four or five times a day and say out loud (if possible), "Right now I'm feeling angry about…" and complete the sentence. Allow yourself to sit for a minute or so with what it feels like to have anger about this subject, without doing anything about it. Yes, it's important to *resolve* anger sometimes, but it's also important to just be able to notice and name it. Sometimes that's enough.

Shared Activity

Since your shared activities are affected by this illness, it's important to acknowledge to one another that anger makes sense and is an appropriate emotion. It may not be time yet to really brainstorm and figure out how to adjust your shared activities, but it's a good place to start to acknowledge that anger is normal and natural, and to communicate that anger to each other so it's not brewing beneath the surface. Try phrasing like "I'm not asking for any type of change yet, and this isn't about guilt tripping, but I just need to acknowledge to you that I'm feeling angry about x, and when the time comes, it's one of the topics that I'd like to negotiate a little better." As the listener, try to not get defensive that your partner is angry. Chronic illness isn't anyone's fault, but it does change everything, and anger about those changes is natural.

Well Partner

In all likelihood, chronic illness has really disrupted the shared activities in your relationship. Particularly if one reason you two got together was a shared activity, and now your partner can't participate, you might feel cheated and have a deep sense of unfairness. You might feel there's no way to express that, because it's not their fault they can't do it, and it might make you sound spoiled or self-centered to be angry about it while your partner is dealing with something so much worse. But if you don't express your disappointment or anger about losing these activities, these feelings will grow into some stubborn long-term resentment. And on top of losing *fun* shared activities, you may not be sharing basic daily activities too—chores, grocery shopping, and so on. You may be burdened with tasks you used to share. Try starting these conversations by saying "None of this is your fault. But I do have feelings about it, and I'm wondering if you can listen to my frustrations like you would listen to a friend." Give yourself a break for feeling angry about these things. Even if you know it's not your partner's fault, it's still okay to feel angry. Anger isn't the same as blame.

Sick Partner

Most of us build a life balanced between the necessary work and chores and the enjoyable activities. Unfortunately, when you're the sick partner, you must use your available energy for the bare necessities of life. Right now, you may not be able to do much—if anything—that you love to do, that makes your life worth living. This will evolve over time, but for now you're likely really angry about the enjoyments denied to you. If these are main ways to connect with your partner, it's a double whammy. And if they then have the gall to be *angry* about the fact you're not doing it—well, you might be seriously enraged. Try to frame your lack of shared activities, both to yourself and to others, as a temporary situation. You can say "I can't go hiking *right now*, but I'm interested in finding a way to do that again at some point." This can help with anger because we all are better at dealing with temporary obstacles than with permanent ones.

EXERCISE: Unhook from Your Anger:

Defusing or coming unhooked from the emotion of anger is key here. Notice anger when it arises, then say to yourself *I notice I'm having the emotion of anger*, or *There's the "anger about sex" story*. If you say to yourself *I'm so pissed about their pressure with sex*, then you and anger are one and the same. Say instead *I notice I'm having the emotion of anger*; then you gain a little distance between you and anger to decide what it's actually about.

Intimacy and Sex

In a monogamous relationship, sex is an activity reserved for the two of you. Even in nonmonogamous relationships, chronic illness may require a renegotiation of terms. It's hard to have open conversations about sex, but it's essential if you want to avoid anger here. What needs are not getting met? If you're the sick partner, try to not get defensive or angry that your partner is suffering sexually. Realize that sex and intimacy are normal human needs, and their suffering does not necessarily mean that you're at fault. You're not. If you're not receptive to hearing about your partner's anger, just remember that they'll still *have* the anger; it'll just be suppressed and is likely to come out in inappropriate ways.

Well Partner

Nothing has happened to your sex drive and desire. You're still the same person with the same needs that you had last week (or whenever your partner was last healthy). The fact that your partner may not be able to engage in sex and intimacy is a particularly dicey prospect, because in most relationships, you can't go elsewhere to meet this need. It can inspire particular anger if you don't actually *believe* your partner when they say they can't engage in sex. As experienced by Juliette in the previous chapter, if the health issue is reproductive and/or invisible, you really only have your partner's say-so that it hurts or they can't do it. If you've had issues with sex and intimacy before and suspect that your partner is using this as an excuse, you might be full of rage. Your life from here on out will be smoother and your relationship healthier if you make a commitment now to *believe your partner.* That's it. Whatever they say about their symptoms, whatever restrictions they might express, just ask yourself: *If I believed my partner 100 percent, how would I respond?* I'm not saying you won't still have anger; you might. But over time you'll shift your intimacy so that you both get your needs met; for now, I'm asking you to believe your partner and trust that you'll find new ways to connect in this area.

At this phase of the process, it's good to get straight that each partner is responsible for their own pleasure (Fogel Mersy and Vencill 2023). Despite our expectations on entering a romantic relationship, it's not entirely your partner's responsibility to meet your needs in this area. You may need to get reintroduced to masturbation or other self-pleasuring activities.

Sick Partner

If you love sex, you might be really mad about the restrictions your condition places on you. But more likely, your partner who isn't sick is pressuring you to have sex. Even if they're not, you may feel guilty about not being able to provide sexual intimacy. There's a particular anger that comes with being asked to participate if you don't feel up to it. Your partner isn't just being a jerk—(well, hopefully not!)—they're a healthy person with a healthy need for sex, and they're dependent on you to meet this need. The more compassion you can have for your partner's situation, the easier it'll be to talk about and negotiate this issue. Even if you're in a nonmonogamous relationship, not being able to participate in sex might disrupt the way your relationships previously worked, and you might be feeling left out or jealous. This is entirely normal as you navigate having to renegotiate these agreements. Fogel Mersy and Vencill state in their book *Desire* that "willingness may be the most important part of your sexual response, not desire or orgasm" (2023, p. 15). Remember that your willingness to at least talk about these issues will go a long way.

EXERCISE: Practice Believing Your Sick Partner

Notice whether any part of your anger focuses on doubting or not believing your partner. Because most chronic illness isn't visible, it's easy to fall into the trap of feeling like your partner *looks* fine and therefore they must *feel* fine. Of course there are people who exaggerate or make up symptoms, but that's relatively rare in the chronic illness community. If your partner says something like "I'm too tired to vacuum" or "It hurts too much to have sex right now," notice if you start feeling anger. Ask yourself if any part of that is tied to doubting or disbelief. Then ask yourself *What if I believed that my partner is being 100 percent truthful about what they are reporting?* If you would respond differently, please do! It's common for the chronically ill to not be believed; you really want to avoid that experience within your intimate relationship.

Friends, Family, and Gatekeeping

Talk together about what's making you angry regarding friends and family. Is it making both of you angry, or just one? Being angry with others in this stage of illness is natural, because others don't anticipate what you'll need or how you'll be feeling. Try to not bash people who are not behaving as you'd wish; just spend some time identifying the issues or actions that create anger in you as a team. This will be helpful when you get to the testing/acceptance phases, so you can start to develop new boundaries. If a situation arises where one of you interacts with friends and family in a way the other finds angering, just notice that anger has come up around it, so you can talk later about potential resolutions.

It's unlikely that you both will have the exact same ideas about who should come and go and when, how others should help and assist you, and what information is okay or not okay. You are two separate individuals who likely have different expectations and boundaries. Often you won't know that something will make you angry until it does. Again, simply note that it didn't work for you, so you can have some open conversation later about potential solutions.

Well Partner

For the healthy partner, there's a temptation to use friends and family as a sounding board for anger. After all, you may feel like you cannot vent your anger toward your partner—because they're sick and upset—but you can let that out with your friends or family. Be careful; how you do this can have lasting consequences. If you vent your anger with friends or family who aren't particularly fond of your partner, they may join you in your anger and later struggle to have a positive relationship with your partner or you as a couple. I advise choosing either a friend who doesn't know your partner (maybe a colleague) or a friend or family member who is mature and emotionally intelligent enough to understand that anger is natural and doesn't necessarily mean that your partner is doing anything wrong. This way, you'll be able to process your angry feelings without damaging relationships. If you don't have anyone like this, a therapist can process these feelings with you.

A healthy partner might also be feeling anger toward outside people or organizations. If you have always enjoyed good health, you might be really angry at doctors or the medical system for not "fixing" your partner. You might be angry at family and friends for not helping, for saying insensitive things, or for interfering too much. It might be your job to protect your partner from them, if they're too sick to do this themself. Understand that expressing your anger toward doctors and friends and family, though often deserved, isn't productive. As in the shock and denial phase, you might need to designate one person to communicate with the rest of the family, ideally a person with whom it's safe to practice saying "I'm angry about…" and let that person instruct the others.

Sick Partner

You may well have some anger toward friends and family. Many of us are not great at dealing with tragedy and illness. People may recommend all kinds of home remedies ("Have you tried apple cider vinegar?"), or just disappear from your life because they don't know what to say. To effectively manage your anger with friends and family, you'll need to get good at defining what is and isn't helpful for you. You're allowed to say "I would rather you not offer any medical solutions; I'm taking care of that," or "Would you come over and just watch funny movies with me, and not talk about my illness at all?" Helping others to understand what's useful to you will help prevent future anger.

As the sick partner, you'll need your partner's help to gatekeep your time and energy. This can create anger because your partner is unlikely to magically create the same boundaries you'd prefer. Your partner might be inviting *everyone* on the planet over to cheer you up, whereas you may want to be left alone. Your partner may be calling every medical specialist in the country, whereas you're more comfortable talking to your primary physician. It's crucial to be crystal clear on what's helpful for you and what isn't helpful for you. Here anger is your friend, because often you can't predict what's going to bug the heck out of you until your partner does it! In that case, you can say to your anger *Oh, thank you for alerting me that doesn't work for me! I'll take care of that so we don't have to be angry about it anymore.*

EXERCISE: Lighten It Up

See if you can find any way to get silly about anger. In the previous chapter, I noted a technique for cognitive defusing: Sing a silly song, or say things in a silly voice. This won't work for every couple, especially since anger is such a raw emotion. But if it's possible to sing "Let it gooooo" at the top of your lungs when your friends send you yet another email about miracle cures, the two of you might find ways to laugh together about things that are so very angering. Right now you're getting used to all of the changes in your relationship; it's no wonder so many things are upsetting. If you can find any way to make these frustrations humorous, it might really help. I don't mean to dismiss or demean anyone's real anger; if either of you feels hurt by the humor, it's not going to work for you. Just see whether you can acknowledge the anger in a way in which disperses it through shared laughter.

EXERCISE: Create an Anger Journal

It's helpful to keep a running list of the things that make you angry. Write them down in an anger journal. For each item, ask yourself if there's a way to clarify what you need from the situation or person that would help resolve the anger. For example, let's say you're enraged because your doctor spent five minutes with you and blew you off. Perhaps you could ask the doctor's office if thirty-minute appointments are available, giving you more time to explain your issues. Or let's say your partner is still expecting you to make dinner every night, and your fatigue is unmanageable. Instead of being angry, you might say "Things have changed for me; I no longer have the stamina to cook every night. Let's make a plan for a dinner rotation or structure that might work better with my situation." Even if there are no immediate solutions, keeping an anger log is a way to get the anger out of you and onto the page.

Moving On

I hope it's been helpful to talk a little about anger. It's such a common emotion in the experience of chronic illness that learning to interact with anger in a healthy way is crucial. Next, we'll look into the bargaining phase, in which a person second-guesses their thoughts or actions or otherwise tries to negotiate or make deals so their new reality might not actually be true. Let's learn how to move through that phase in a healthy way.

Chapter 5

Bargaining Phase

What You Will Learn in This Chapter:

- Feelings of "if only" are a hallmark of the bargaining phase.
- We tend to assign meaning, often spiritual, to bad things that happen to us.
- Feelings of regret and hope are central in this phase, and often different for each partner.
- Other people can be challenging in this phase because they'll offer lots of suggestions.
- Finding your values can help guide what activities and goals you pursue in your wellness journey.
- Your goals and activities may change now that chronic illness is in the picture, but you can still be true to your values.

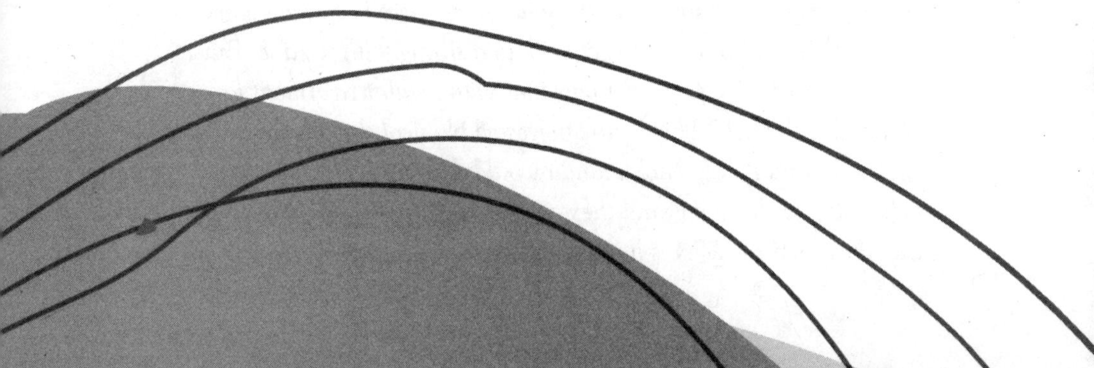

"Yeah, yeah," Juanita says to her friend on the phone, "I know the doctor says that fibromyalgia doesn't have a cure, but there are so many options for treatment; I'm gonna beat this thing." Juanita doesn't like having fibromyalgia, and she's going to get rid of it. She has a plan. She's become a keyboard warrior, researching everything she can about this disease. She just bought a boatload of supplements that are supposed to help, and she made an appointment for transcranial magnetic stimulation. Next week, she's got a reiki appointment set up, and then she's getting a massage. If all of this doesn't work, she has some other ideas up her sleeve—tai chi, acupuncture, maybe even ketamine.

Tim hears Juanita on the phone and rolls his eyes. Juanita says she has this thing called fibromyalgia, but Tim isn't even sure it's real. He thinks she doesn't feel well because her diet is terrible and she never exercises. She's somewhat of a hypochondriac. Tim doesn't really approve of the amount of money she's spending on all of these experimental treatments with no scientific backing or hope of working. If only Juanita would just do the basics in taking care of herself—cut out the sweets, take more walks, and get a good night's sleep. That's what Tim does, and he feels fine.

Mohammad's doctor tells him that he has degenerative disk disease in his spine and that's why his back hurts all the time. Mohammad isn't interested in hearing what the doctor has to say in terms of treatment, because he knows what the cause is. He has been lax in his faithfulness to Islam since he moved to America, and Allah is punishing him for it. Mohammad feels that if he gets back to the mosque and his daily prayer routine, Allah will bless him with a pain-free life.

Asmaa agrees that she and Mohammad have been remiss in their faith; she also wants to get back to a strong faith routine. But she doesn't see why they can't pair that with regular treatment for Mohammed's back. The doctor suggested physical therapy and joint injections, and if only Mohammad would do that, he could have some relief for his pain, and they could go back to enjoying life the way they used to. Why is he so stubborn?

The Lay of the Land

"If only" is the hallmark of the bargaining phase. In this phase, we try to find anything and everything that'll make things go back to how they were before. Now, there's nothing wrong with looking for treatments and cures when you don't feel well. But the sense in this phase is somewhat frenetic. Often in the bargaining phase, there isn't a systematic, logical plan; it's more like being in a huge room full of bouncing balls (the balls being cures, ideas, treatments) and just grabbing whatever comes your way. Observers might feel like the sick person and their partner are just flitting from thing to thing in search of a solution.

Becoming chronically ill sparks something in most of us: regret. *If only I hadn't eaten so many cheeseburgers. If only I had exercised more. If only I hadn't climbed up on that ladder. If only I hadn't gotten that surgery.* It goes on and on. You imagine some fateful decision you made that resulted in this terrible condition, and if only you could go back and change it, things would be different.

Sometimes it's true that decisions you've made have had some sort of effect on your current illness. But in most cases you've been living much the same as everyone around you, making the best decisions you can in tough circumstances, and the wheel of fate just landed on you. And even when there *is* something you could have done, the reality is that you're here now, and no amount of regret will change things.

Diagnosis may also spur magical thinking: If only you can find that one thing that will cure you, everything will be all right. Most of us expect that when there's a problem, we can just fix it. Everything can be fixed, right? Because this is how we think, we apply this same philosophy to our illness. If you can just find the fix, things can go back to how they were before. There are whole industries that rely on this type of thinking—and algorithms that will support these industries once you start researching a cure.

In this phase more than the others, spiritual beliefs seem to come into play. Regardless of your faith background, if any, most of us do interpret what happens in our life based on what we believe about how the universe works. You might believe in God, Jesus, Allah, Krishna, karma, or something else. But often in the bargaining phase, you assign meaning to what's happened to you based on what you believe in, which can lead to a lot of "if onlys" or plans about how to fix this result. Either God has abandoned you, you're being punished, or you've created this result through some action you have or haven't taken. If you go back to church, make that wrong right, spend more time doing charitable work in your community, or do some sort of supplication, things will improve. Spiritual beliefs are incredibly important to many people, and there's nothing wrong with that—they can bring you comfort and help you make sense of the world. But in this phase such beliefs can result in a lot of magical thinking, such as believing if you do *x*, it will resolve *y*.

It's not that there aren't things, such as prayer or restorative practices, that may work to help you feel better in whatever illness you're immersed in. But with chronic illnesses for which there are no cures, although you can hope for help and relief, there are usually no quick, permanent fixes. In the bargaining phase, you may get lost in regret and magical thinking, and this can really drive a wedge between partners, especially if they view this phase differently.

Communication and Emotions

With the emotion of regret so central during the bargaining phase, both partners may feel it, depending on what led to the diagnosis. Some people are practical (*we're here now, so what's the point in thinking about what we did or didn't do?*), while others tend more toward ruminating (*I can't believe I did/didn't do that—how can I ever move past this?*)—and often these two types are partnered up.

It's important to communicate about feelings of regret. Not to dwell on the unchangeable past, or to wallow in it, but just so the feeling can move through you and then disperse. Try saying "I know we can't change the past, but I think if we can sit down and talk about our regrets, with the intent to let them go, it might be helpful."

And then there's the emotion of hope—hope that something can help. Hope is great and necessary, but it's important that it not be unrealistic. If your hope makes your partner roll their eyes, or you scoff at your partner's hope, you'll soon find yourselves disconnected from each other. It's a good idea to sit down and talk about what outcome you would each hope for, and how you imagine you'll get there. Are your ideas in line with each other? Vastly different? Perhaps you can prioritize what actions you'll take, respecting both of your opinions and ideas.

Shared Activity

Because partners often diverge in the bargaining phase, sometimes the desire for a cure results in very individualistic behavior. After all, if you're the one who is sick and you want to try acupuncture, biofeedback, and physical therapy, those are not necessarily activities your partner needs or wants to do themself. It can therefore feel very lonely to spend your time developing new activities without your partner's joining you.

One way to avoid that loneliness is to go together to appointments, even if your partner isn't participating. That way, your partner knows what you're experiencing and can enter into conversations about it. Or set aside time to talk about your new activities and—if you're the well partner—ask questions and be interested.

In the bargaining phase, the well partner may pressure the other to engage in previous activities, like hiking or working out, because they feel that this will alleviate symptoms or even effect a cure. The sick partner may feel like they can no longer do these activities, and the insistence that they do can become a problem. Toni Bernhard (Bernhard 2010, p. 122) recommends practicing "wise inaction," and both partners will need to commit to this. This means being attuned to your body's wisdom and your current circumstances and sometimes deciding that the wisest thing you can do is rest.

Intimacy and Sex

In the bargaining stage, sexual intimacy can go one of two ways, depending on whether you or your partner feel that sex will be restorative and healing or you feel that sex will hinder or harm your healing. In chronic illnesses that involve the reproductive system, like endometriosis, one partner may feel that continuing to have sex would be helpful, and the other may disagree. A client of mine was told by her doctor that continuing to have sex would be helpful in the long run, but having sex was still painful for her. Her partner was fixated on what the doctor said, constantly encouraging her to participate so that she could get better. But my client felt that her pain took precedence over whatever potential future benefit there might be in engaging in sex now. Her partner shouldn't have put her in the middle of his own bargaining ("if we have more sex, she will feel less pain in the long term"). Both partners should remember that intimacy and sex is important in relationships, so they need to continue to have conversations about how to involve it in their relationship in a way that both parties are comfortable with.

On the other hand, someone like Asmaa, in the chapter's introductory anecdotes, may feel like Mohammed should avoid sex because he might hurt his back, while Mohammed might feel like his back pain matters less than the connection he would be losing without sex. Sometimes you may want to dissociate yourself from any kind of weakness surrounding your illness; you may feel like if only you can fake it until you make it, things will turn around.

Friends, Family, and Gatekeeping

In this phase, friends and family might really challenge you. Once you have some condition that causes you to feel unwell, everyone you know will email you, forward articles, and tell you about every bizarre internet cure they have ever come across. Your friends and family have their own "if onlys," and they'll truly believe that if only you did this cleanse or that treatment, you'd be better. This can be very stressful for both partners.

In your own desire to find relief, you may fall into the trap of being initially interested in forwarded information—and there isn't anything wrong with this. Others can be a source of good information, perhaps information that you haven't come across yourself. But ultimately, you may find yourself overwhelmed by other people's insistence that you should just do *x* or *y* to feel better.

You may have to set some boundaries around what kind of information you're open to, and what kind of responses your family and friends should expect from you when they give you information. If you say "Please don't forward me any information about my illness unless I ask for feedback," people might still do it, but you can just continue to politely yet firmly set this boundary until it sticks.

A roller coaster cycle can develop during this phase: You become excited whenever a friend or doctor suggests a new treatment, only to become despondent when that treatment does not live up to the hype. After you've gone through this cycle a few times, you may want to come up with a system for receiving and trying out new information.

Everyone does this differently, depending on their condition and how much they get emotionally involved in suggestions. Some people may want to tell others that they want only the information they ask for, and no unsolicited advice. Others may want to keep lists of suggestions and look at them only when they feel emotionally prepared to consider the information.

Reflection Questions

1. Have you had self-criticism around anything you might have done that you perceive could have caused your illness? If so, are you able to adopt a more self-compassionate dialogue?
2. Have you tried any alternative treatments to try to obtain a cure? How did you feel after doing this?
3. Have you argued with your partner about the cost and/or time involved in any of these treatments?

Coping with Bargaining

As a team, you can decide what kind of bargaining activities you're open to in general. Do you want others to suggest treatment options? What will you do with this information together? Do you want to visit alternative doctors and healers to see what they have to suggest? How will you decide together which options to pursue? It's good to ask these questions and have a policy as a team—rather than operating independently—so that you don't become lost in all the well-meaning suggestions, or start arguing about which options you're pursuing.

ACT Skill: Finding Values

When you're caught up in regret from the past or the multitude of healing options, it's helpful to have guidance in determining how to proceed. The ACT skill of defining and becoming very clear on your values—both as an individual and as a couple—is such a guide. Defining and being led by your values is *always* helpful, especially during the bargaining phase.

I'm always surprised at how few people have any idea what their values are or have ever given this much thought. Most of us have some vague idea. But vague ideas don't usually work to drive behavior. Some people—often religious individuals—have been handed a set of values they are supposed to believe in. But many haven't really thought through whether they actually resonate with those values. Regardless of your values background—religious or otherwise—identifying your values can help you not only derive meaning from this period of your illness but also decide what avenues align most closely with that meaning. For example, if your spiritual faith *is* a value for you, you might choose a prayer group. But if it's not, you might choose something like a mindfulness retreat.

When it comes to understanding values, another complication is that sometimes people view values as synonymous with goals or actions, even though they're not the same thing. Luckily, ACT provides some specific defining features of values and ways to determine what yours are. Values are what you most care about, what you want your life to be about, and what you want to stand for. They are your "chosen life direction" (Harris 2009, p. 189). Goals are items you can complete and tick off on a list (like getting a degree or completing a marathon); values are more about overarching qualities. Values are always available to us, even when we aren't meeting particular related goals. The table offers some examples that apply to chronic illness.

Value	Goal
Be curious and open	Try acupuncture to see if it helps
Care for my body	Sleep eight hours a night
Be centered and calm	Learn to meditate

If you have a value of caring for your body, you might establish a goal of sleeping for eight hours a night. However, that might prove challenging. Perhaps your pain keeps you awake, or a medication you're on prevents good sleep, so you need to readjust the goal. Or if you consistently achieve that goal, you may need to set more goals that help you live your value of caring for your body. But no matter how your goals change or adjust, the *value* of caring for your body remains constant. You'll carry that value for the long haul and express it in many different ways.

In the context of chronic illness, it helps to establish values you can be true to even if your condition never changes. Success and meaning in life come from living your values, and you can still do that even if you're sick. The *goals* might change, but the values don't have to.

So, for example, if your value is to contribute in meaningful ways to the world, you may have done all kinds of active things before you got sick. Maybe you cleaned up waterways, went to marches, or campaigned actively for candidates you believe in. You might feel despondent that you can't act on your values in these specific ways any more. However, you don't have to abandon that value; you need only to adjust the *ways* you act on it. But perhaps now you do the background organizing for the march, or call voters instead of going door to door.

Knowing your values will help you in the bargaining phase because they will dictate your goals and actions and keep you from frenetically bouncing from thing to thing. If you have really defined values about how you spend your money, you'll make different decisions on how you spend it on healing. If you value productivity, you may need to redefine rest as a productive activity in the healing process. If you value animal rights, you may not take certain supplements that don't honor that value, even if your best friend's sister says they're miraculous.

Values will keep you centered when the ideas you find on the internet and others present to you would otherwise have you in a whirlwind of bargaining and confusion. And defining your values and living according to them can keep you from feeling like your life is "over" or that nothing matters now that life have changed. I have a client (who gave me permission to share) who is paralyzed and in a wheelchair as a result of a medical accident. Before his accident, he always got what he wanted, sometimes at the expense of other people's feelings. He claimed to value having a loving community, but his actions didn't always align with that value. But since his accident, he's started to sync his actions with that value, and I admire the circle of love and support that he and his wife have developed.

His ex-wife is close friends with his current wife. He still sits on the stage with his band even though he can no longer play guitar, and people come out specifically to see him and give him a hug. Sometimes we talk about whether he would've been able to garner this loving, supportive circle had his life not turned out this way. He doesn't think so. Of course, it would be nice to have achieved this value in some other, less traumatizing way. But he's living much more in tune with his values now than he did before the accident, and this helps him accept his new reality.

Reflection Questions

1. Have you ever thought about your life values? Do you think it will be easy to identify these, or a challenge?
2. Do you think you and your partner have the same values in general, or different ones?

Chapter Summary Points

- Often people engage in magical thinking that “if only” they’d done something different or “if only” they could do some magical cure, they’d be well again.
- Partners have different versions of this thinking, and communication is important to understand where each partner is coming from.
- Other people may need to be managed in this phase, because people who love you tend to let you know about every possible cure they hear about. Setting boundaries here is crucial.
- Values can help guide your goals and activities in this phase, so you pursue things that really align with who you want to be in life.
- Even though you’re sick, you can still create a life of meaning that aligns with your values, although it may look different from your former vision.

Moving On

In the next chapter, we'll discuss some specific ways to find your values and create a life that's true to them, regardless of your current circumstances. I offer a list of potential values that have come up for clients in my practice. Some are opposites, and some may conflict with others. Values are very personal; there are no right or wrong value systems when it comes to healing. Think about your "if onlys"—how you've responded to what has happened to you. We'll look over those values and consider whether any could potentially help you in finding your way forward. And we'll talk about specific issues you may each have in the bargaining phase and how to work productively with these concerns.

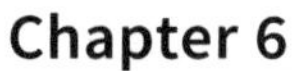

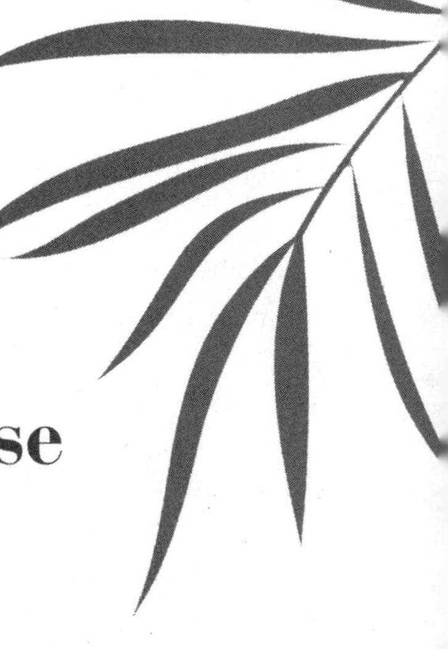

Chapter 6

Tools for the Bargaining Phase

In this phase of chronic illness, you tend to be either lost in regret about what you did or didn't do, or so hopeful about different potential cures that you're being swayed by every scrap of information that comes your way. Partners often feel vastly different from each other in this phase, so communication will be particularly important to support one another and prioritize your next steps.

How You May Be Feeling

This can be a very tumultuous stage of illness for each of you individually and both of you as a team. You might both have *If only I had* or *If only we had* thoughts, and these might go in very different directions. You might both be intensely searching for a way forward, ways that also may be vastly different in method and style. Sometimes partners are impatient with each other's choices, so it's really important to be able to come together in this phase without judgment for feeling differently. It's okay to differ in your feelings about both your past and your future direction. But to thrive as partners, you need to find ways to understand and support each other.

Well Partner

This is a difficult phase for you, in terms of both your own feelings and watching what your partner may be doing in their quest to feel better. You might have a lot of unexpressed feelings about how your partner got to this place in their life, but you are reluctant to accuse your partner of doing harmful things or not doing things they should have done. Or maybe you *do* accuse them, and *that's* not going well! You understand that you're here now, but what do you do with all these feelings?

Sick Partner

I get it. When you're sick with a condition for which there is no cure—and often very little effective help from the medical community—you turn to the internet. There's a wealth of information out there from all the people with experience. Entire industries thrive on the promise of making you feel better—and that's not always a bad thing. There's nothing wrong with researching, reading, and gathering information that might help you. It's vital to have hope for the future. The problem for your significant other is that you're the one living in your body, but you also must consider the time, money, and attention that may be getting siphoned off from what used to belong to you both as partners.

Communication and Emotions

It's important to be able to communicate both how you regard past choices and also how you should proceed from here. If you two have vastly different viewpoints, that's okay, but it won't help to judge one another or refuse to hear how the other person feels. This is confusing for everyone—you're caught in an illness that no one has the answers for, and now you're also swirling in that confusion as a couple.

One way to learn to calmly listen to one another without judgment is to make sure you're having conversations in a calm moment, rather than when you've been activated by something your partner has done that you aren't happy with. Listening, understanding, and validating aren't the same as agreement, so you can listen and try to understand your partner's point of view without necessarily sharing it. Try saying "I don't feel the same, but I can see how this feels from your point of view, and if I were in your position, I might feel like that too." Try to keep an open mind about their thoughts and feelings so you can truly understand where they're coming from. It helps to set the ground rules for these conversations in advance—something like "I know we feel differently, but it's important that we really understand how each of us feels. So let's talk about it, not to solve anything, but to just see if we can get a handle on where we each are."

Well Partner

It's important to not internalize and suppress your negative feelings. This is like shaking up a soda bottle; at some point, all that fizz is going to come leaking out. You may have many feelings: anger for past choices, frustration at current choices, and helplessness from being unable to find anything helpful. Your relationship might be such that you can carve out a safe space and time for you both to share your differing emotions on these topics. But in this phase it might be useful to have someone else to confide in about how you're feeling—a person who's not judgmental of your partner and their choices, but can be a sounding board so you can sort out how you're feeling about all of it without critique. This could be a helping professional or a support group.

In addition, you likely need to talk about money and finances. Most partners already have some disagreements about finances, and this phase, when your partner is eager to try anything that will help, may put a strain on your financial plan. In the US healthcare system, most healing modalities are expensive, and many of them are not covered by traditional insurance. Your partner is ill and wants to feel better, so they may not be as concerned about how much everything is costing. But you may need to communicate your concern about how this may affect your finances. Try to do this in a way that allows room for your partner to try things they want to try, maybe just suggesting a different pacing that your budget can accommodate. Try saying "I really want you to pursue treatment in any way you can. But I also want us to be financially sound. Can we make a plan together on how and when to try each thing so that our budget doesn't suffer?"

Sick Partner

It can be mightily frustrating when you think you've found an approach that might help you—and your partner shuts it down. You might just feel like your partner doesn't approve, or they may actually tell you that these approaches are unproven and a waste of money. Or maybe they're right alongside you looking at all kinds of cures. Either way, you're feeling desperate for anything you can find that offers relief or improvement. That makes total sense; you have every right to explore options. Just understand that whatever your diagnosis, this process can be exhausting and often disappointing. It's a marathon, not a sprint, so pace yourself. Try to develop a sustainable approach to exploring treatments. For example, you might list every treatment option you've come across and organize them into phases or cost/time allotments. At the same time, try to keep the lines of communication open with your partner, explaining what you're learning and why you think particular avenues might be worth exploring. It really smooths the way if you acknowledge the strain, perhaps by saying "I know we don't have unlimited funds, and I also really want to pursue this. Can we talk about a way to fit this into our budget?"

EXERCISE: Assess Your Feelings

It's important to assess how you feel about what your partner is doing and saying. Look back at the feelings chart in chapter 1; can you identify how you're feeling now? Take some time to journal your honest feelings, even if you wouldn't necessarily share them with your partner. Then decide how you might productively share your concerns with your partner at the right time.

The following prompts can get you started. These are of course just a small sample of possible emotions. Your feelings are valid and important—they just might be different from your partner's feelings.

- Are you annoyed?
- Are you worried about the money being spent?
- Are you jumping on the bandwagon of every potential remedy?
- Are you mad that you're getting shut down when you're excited about something?
- Are you frustrated that they're dwelling on "if onlys" that you can't go back and change?

Shared Activity

In this phase it's important to find shared activity but also to respect the individual activities you each need to pursue on this healing journey. In the exercises, I'll have you come up with some things that you can pursue as a team. But understand that you're on two different journeys, even as you travel together. The sick partner is looking for healing from a medical condition for which there are no (or very few) reliable treatments. And the well partner also has a healing journey, from the additional stress of caring for an ill partner, taking over responsibilities and tasks they can't handle, or even just financially supporting this process. So the well partner also may need to explore and add some healing modalities. Doing these things together can be helpful for both of you, but don't discount time alone, as long as there is space to communicate about what you're learning and to support one another.

Even if you're sharing some activities, they're almost always in service of healing, because that's the focus of this phase. But it's exhausting to pursue healing 24/7, so consider reserving time together for pure fun and pleasure, not focused on the illness or healing. Doing a puzzle, watching movies, or playing a game can be connecting and give you a break from the heaviness of searching for better health.

Well Partner

In this phase, partners often diverge in terms of shared activities. Many of the treatments and hopeful approaches that a sick partner engages in are solitary activities. It's true, you could join your partner in a tai chi or yoga class or retreat, but many modalities—acupuncture, hyperbaric oxygen chambers, bodywork, and the like—are intended for the sick person to pursue on their own. It might be worth exploring what kinds of healthy, restful, and relaxing activities you can engage in together. If your partner is pursuing individual approaches, maybe you can at least have a shared activity of researching and discussing possibilities before your partner goes off to try them on their own. Remember that you too have a lot of tension and strong emotion—many of these healing activities could be good for you as well.

Caregiving is well known to be very stressful, and most of us have heard the caution that too often caregivers ultimately break down before their sick partners do. Pay some attention to your stress level as well, and think about potential new activities that might replenish your energy and provide renewal. These don't have to be the same activities your partner is doing.

Sick Partner

If you're deep into remedy explorations, you might be getting impatient with your partner's wanting to spend time together. It might seem like time's a-wastin', and you don't have the time to be off having fun when you could be doing more research on your condition. If your partner is open to alternative healing modalities, try to include them in your research and experiments. For example, if you're going down to your local spa to try infrared therapy, see if your partner wants to come too. As long as what you're trying isn't harmful, you might find things that you both enjoy doing. You're going to need a healthy partner to support you, so try to encourage your partner to engage in healing activities as well, even if they aren't the same ones you're doing. Make room in the schedule for them to do things—like hiking with a friend or going to the gym—that'll take care of their health and well-being as well.

EXERCISE: Make an Activities List

I don't know about you, but if someone asks me "What do you want to do right now?" I can never think of a thing, even though I often have things I want to do! So I have even my healthy couple clients make a running list of activities that they might like to try.

For this exercise, each of you sit down separately and make a list of activities you might like to do. You may need to get creative and look at local magazines or pursue ideas on the internet. When you each have a list, sit down and compare them. Anything on both your lists can go on the master list. Activities you've listed that your partner hasn't listed can be negotiated, or you can alternate those activities, as long as they are feasible for the sick partner. If finances are an issue, it can also be useful to separate activities by cost. Once you have a master list, you can put it somewhere visible, then continue to add to the list as activities come to mind or become possible.

Create categories like:

- Activities I want to do by myself
- Activities I'd like us to do together
- Healing activities
- Fun activities
- Activities that require more time (a day or a weekend)
- Activities we can do with small pockets of time

Intimacy and Sex

As we're talking about exploring healing on this journey, note that sometimes sex and intimacy can be used in an unhealthy way, whether it's pushing for sex as a tool to feel better or avoiding sex and intimacy altogether. I know you're exhausted and trying to make room for just what you think might be helpful to you. And while the power of touch and connection should be one of the healing activities that's always in your toolbox, sometimes you may feel on very different pages during this phase, and communication may be fraught with disagreement. Leaning in to sensual or comforting touch is an area where you might be able to find rest and agreement, as long as there's agreement about how you're approaching it. Try defining a period of time with parameters, like "We are going to lie together on the bed, skin to skin, for twenty minutes, but it's not going to develop into anything further" so that you both feel safe and comfortable.

Well Partner

Often, sex will wane in this phase because the sick partner doesn't see it as a healing activity and their attention and focus is on what might be helpful to them. You may find yourself pressuring your partner for more sexual intimacy, perhaps just because you need it or perhaps because you honestly feel it'll help them feel better. Consent is key, and lack of consent will harm your sex life in the long term, so it's important to find out what does and doesn't feel good for your partner. Simple touch is often good for both of you, and lying skin to skin or just snuggling is an activity that feels good and is also low-energy.

You may be struggling quite a bit at this point with less sex or no sex in your relationship. Try to make the focus on the healing properties of human connection and touch, and ask your partner in what ways touch and closeness could feel healing and good to them. Be patient; this is a process! It's okay to say "I'm really struggling here, but I can handle it," but also maybe "It would really help me if we could touch more, in ways that feel doable for you. Can we brainstorm about that?"

I suggest you read a book like *The Ultimate Guide to Sex and Disability* (Kaufman, Silverberg, and Odette 2003). Your partner will appreciate your taking the time to learn about the difficulties, and it may open up avenues for discussion.

Sick Partner

Sex and intimacy can get caught up in bargaining, whether you pursue sex relentlessly to feel pleasure or swear off of it in order to heal. Try not to think rigidly about intimacy; there are lots of creative options. Intimacy and sex might seem like a waste of time to you right now; after all, you're trying to find a way to feel better and get through the day. Or you might be feeling so poorly that sex is the only thing you can think of that you can still associate with your body and pleasure. Remember that sexual intimacy is more than just intercourse. There are many ways of physical sharing that are sensual and feel good—and you probably have enough energy to enjoy with your partner—as long as you agree on boundaries. Be clear on what you can and can't do at this point, and assure your partner that you still love them and are trying to get yourself back to a point where you can be fully sexual again.

It's widely known that healthy relationships that are emotionally and physically connected contribute to good health. So don't discount just spending sensual time with your partner (even if it's not sexual) and view that as time spent on your own personal healing.

EXERCISE: Listing the Possibilities

Find a time to sit down together when life is calm (it does happen!) to talk about what outcomes you're hoping for. Take turns describing your understanding about intimacy vis-a-vis the illness right now, where you'd like to get to ideally, and steps you would take to get there. The well partner will need to try to not get offended if the sick partner doesn't seem to share the same desperation or urgency to resolve intimacy issues; the sick partner may need to manage their exasperation at the inventive ideas their partner may want to try. Try to compile a list of all possible solutions or experiments you'd like to try, then see if you can prioritize actions for going forward. One area of exploration is *sensate focus*, a series of exercises you can find on the internet or in books such as *Desire: An Inclusive Guide to Navigating Libido Differences in Relationships* (Fogel Mersy and Vencill 2023). Here are some potential ideas:

- Lie together, making eye contact, with simple touch—perhaps a hug.
- Practice touching with a focus on temperature, pressure, and texture, with chests and genitals off limits.
- Have the well partner engage in self-stimulation with the sick partner simply present.

Friends, Family, and Gatekeeping

Boundaries is the name of the game with other people during this phase of your illness journey. You're looking for remedies and cures, and everyone around you is also hoping that things can "get back to normal." If you're open to trying alternatives, others may feel invited to forward you every bizarre and miraculous cure they hear about. Often they have no real understanding of your condition, and some suggestions may not apply or even be harmful. Decide as a team how you want to handle this. Will one or both of you set boundaries with others about how you want to be communicated with? Do you want to view this information as it comes in, or set aside a time each week to sift through the suggestions? Will you do this together or separately? It's easy to go off on individual tangents in this phase, and we want to keep you working as a team.

Gatekeeping here is important: While you're deciding what kind of information you want to receive from other people, explore whether you or your partner will set the boundaries. Obviously you'll need to set your own boundaries with your own friends, but with shared family and friends, you'll need to decide if one or both of you will speak for your relationship. In any case, you'll want to send a unified message.

Well Partner

Your friends and family will give you lots of advice and information. Depending on whether or not you're open to ideas, they might be giving you loads of suggestions or dismissing any ideas you have for cures and remedies. You might become super impatient with all of this and find yourself snapping or otherwise responding impatiently. Try taking some time just for yourself to figure out your feelings on receiving information. Your partner may feel differently, of course, but it's important to know how *you* feel about all of it.

Sick Partner

You might be asking everyone you know for ideas, or you might just be downright sick of their silly ideas, or something in between. In this phase, you may become so obsessed with research and healing that it's all you want to talk about. Supportive family and friends may become obsessed too, which might mean they forward every single idea they find on social media. You might love this or hate it; everyone is different. Don't be afraid to tell people what works for you and what doesn't. They don't know until you tell them. Also, if it helps to have your partner be the one to respond, make sure your partner knows this—and also what you do and don't want them to say. Your partner can really help you, but you need to be on the same page.

EXERCISE: Find Your Individual Values

Look at the table of values here and choose three to five that are particularly important to you. (Get a longer list at newharbinger.com/56081.) When making your selection, imagine looking back on your life at age eighty. What could you be able to say about who you were? Is that different now than it was before chronic illness came along?

SHORT LIST OF VALUES

Mind	**Body**	**Relationship**	**Action**
Flexibility	Self-care	Connection	Contribution
Humor	Self-control	Intimacy	Fun
Authenticity	Sensuality	Reciprocity	Creativity
Compassion	Well-being	Trust	Persistence

Once you've decided on your values, think about how you and your partner can use shared activity to act on them. Create a couple of related goals that are doable now, even under these circumstances. For example, if you have the value of creativity, you could set the goal to attend an art class with your partner; if a value is justice, you and your partner could volunteer for a political or social cause you care about.

Think, too, about how living your values may have changed since you became sick. How did living out those values look before this happened? Did you have goals then that you can't accomplish now? How would it look to keep those values, but reassess how to live them out under new circumstances?

EXERCISE: Finding Shared Values

Values will guide this discussion just as they will guide you as individuals. What are your values as a unit? Think about celebrating your fiftieth anniversary.

- What do you want people to be able to say about you as a couple?
- Is this different now from before your chronic illness?
- As a team, what do you want to be known for?
- How do the experiments from the previous exercise line up with these values?
- Does pursuing any of these remedies conflict with any values?
- Do any of the activities line up directly with your values?

You may need to resort to your earlier list, based on the values you've identified as a team.

Moving On

Dealing with regret from the past, managing how you hope for the future as partners—it's a real challenge. Hopefully you've been able to move through this phase and find some ways to align your values as you each navigate this new reality. However, your chosen activities and goals may mean some remedies and cures *don't* work, leaving you back at square one, or sometimes even worse off than you were before. That's part of the process, but can sometimes lead to real despair. In the next two chapters, we will talk about the sadness and depression that can sometimes result from pursuing health.

Chapter 7

Depression Phase

What You Will Learn in This Chapter:

- Depression can happen at any point, even though I've put it here after *bargaining*.
- Depression is the phase you may find yourself cycling through the most often.
- Depression is a completely natural response to your life's falling apart and your being unable to find any help.
- Suicidal thoughts are also natural; however, if these thoughts are more than transitory, you need to pursue treatment.
- There are two parts of you—the you that is thinking, and the you that can observe you thinking.
- Your depression is happening to you; it's not you.
- Understanding there's more to you than your symptoms of depression can help you remember who you really are.

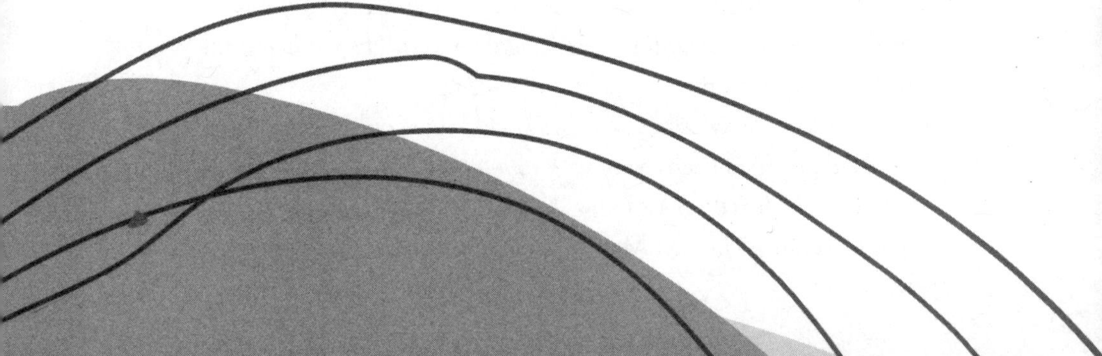

Sara is lying in bed, wearing a sleep mask, the curtains closed. She feels like she can't tolerate any movement whatsoever and wishes she could just lie there indefinitely. A lot of it is physical—she got COVID early on, before vaccines, and hasn't been able to recover. She's been diagnosed with postural orthostatic tachycardia syndrome (POTS) and has myalgic encephalomyelitis/chronic fatigue syndrome (ME/CFS) symptoms, and she hasn't been able to find any help. She's been told she should exercise more, that it's all in her head, and that she's faking it entirely. She's gone to a long COVID clinic and tried all kinds of vitamin regimens and even hyperbaric oxygen. Last month she was in a Paxlovid trial, with high hopes it would help her. But it didn't. She feels like she's out of options, and depression has set in.

Sara's partner, Heidi, gets it. Her hopes have been dashed too, multiple times. But she feels like science is moving forward all the time, and so many people are working on this issue now because of its exposure in the news. Heidi feels like it's just a matter of time before someone comes up with something that will work for Sara; they need to just stay positive. She cognitively knows what depression is like, but she hasn't experienced it and can't really understand why Sara can't just snap out of it. Wouldn't getting up and doing things be better than just lying there?

Lewis has degenerative disk disorder, with constant back pain. Unlike Sara, he got to the depressed phase right off the bat. He's had depression off and on for his entire life, so this isn't anything new. He went to the doctor expecting to find something strategic they could do to relieve his pain, but found out there are really not very many treatment options; he's going to be living with some kind of pain for the rest of his life. Lewis isn't motivated to explore any of the available options, including nonmedical options. He just heard the doctor say he'd be living in pain and gave up.

Lewis's wife, Mercy, is mad as heck. How could Lewis just give up like that? She's been living with him a long time, so she knows this is how he deals with things, but she thought he'd at least explore options before giving up. Mercy knows it'll be hard enough living with someone who's in constant pain, but now she has to live with a depressed person, too! It's enough to make her depressed and feel like giving up. Where does a person even go from here?

The Lay of the Land

In this book, I've put depression after bargaining, because often depression kicks in after a frenzy of trying everything available and discovering that nothing is the fix you hoped for. But honestly, depression can set in at any phase of chronic illness, and it might be the phase you cycle through most often. Also, each partner is likely to cycle through depression, perhaps for different reasons. As it becomes clear that things might never be the same, both partners lose dreams they had for their future.

Most of my clients have been told at one time or another that their illness is "all in their head." Obviously, it isn't—yet almost every client I have with chronic illness *also* has some sort of depression or anxiety. I mean, it makes sense, right? How could you *not* be depressed or anxious from time to time, if not regularly? That's not to say it's the *cause* of your illness, but it's a reality and also needs to be treated. Many of my clients resist medication options for depression (or anxiety) because they don't want doctors to pass off symptoms they're having as a mental health issue. This is a *valid* concern. However, it does break my heart to see some people not receiving treatment that could help them because of the way the system works. Depression in chronic illness is common, real, and deserves its own treatment.

Here are a few quotes from chronic illness memoirs:

> I had a sense that my battery was drained. I was coming up against a physical reality that conflicted with my assumptions that I would, by now, be on an upward trajectory…I found the burden of positivity weighed on me after just a few days. What was I supposed to do with my fears, my darker thoughts?...the annihilating absence of language, the impossibility of finding a story to tell about the blankness that confronted me day after day, the chasm between me and other humans. (O'Rourke 2023)

> I was starting to spiral downward, again, and when I looked into my affirmation-adorned mirror, I could see the desperation creeping into my eyes…This time when they told me I was depressed and needed medications and psychiatric intervention, I sagged in my chair but did not argue. I wasn't depressed. I was destroyed… Wanting to escape this crushing predicament isn't a defect—it's the natural response. Of course we want out. Of course it's too difficult to bear. Of course we do everything we can to scale the walls, to get back to life as we knew it. (Ramey 2020)

> With the cloud came, for the first time in my life, a suicidal current in my thoughts—temporary like all my symptoms and therefore survivable, but still a repeated pulse of *just kill yourself, just kill yourself, just kill yourself* that lasted anywhere from a few minutes to an hour before it fled…But when the crisis simply continues without resolution, when the illness grinds on and on and on—well, then a curtain tends to fall, because there isn't an obvious way to integrate that kind of struggle into the realm of everyday life. (Douthat 2021)

I'd like to talk a bit about suicidality or suicidal ideation, since it was mentioned in the preceding quote. When you're in an extremely painful situation, and there doesn't seem to be any resolution in sight, it's natural to feel depressed and, for some of you, to turn toward thoughts of suicide in order to cope with the unending misery. For many of my clients, this takes the form of "I just don't want to [or can't] do this anymore," not because they're planning to take their life, but because that's a natural feeling to have in this circumstance. For others, the thoughts may be more actively suicidal, but transitory and temporary, like what Douthat experienced. If you fall into these two camps, I encourage you to find someone you can talk to openly about these feelings. That may not be your partner—this kind of talk is scary for many people, and sometimes it may be a therapist that you'll need in order to fully process these desperate but normal feelings. It's entirely normal to have these thoughts, and there's no shame in expressing them to the right person. As long as these thoughts are transitory and temporary, you need not worry about their indicating something wrong—it's entirely natural to feel this way in your circumstances.

Many people are reluctant to express these thoughts to a counselor because they worry that they'll get admitted to a psychiatric facility. I assure you that almost all mental health professionals are trained for and comfortable talking about suicidal thoughts. Admission to a psychiatric hospital can occur, but only when there's intent and a plan. You can safely discuss suicidal *thoughts* with a mental health professional without worrying about hospitalization.

Some of you may take these thoughts a bit further, experiencing thoughts of suicide that don't go away and even develop into planning. While it's entirely natural to have these feelings, you don't need to suffer in this way. You must have a mental health professional help you to deal with the thoughts and feelings, and this is the time to consider appropriate medication.

If you're the partner of the suicidal person, and they express suicidal intent with a plan, you must call 911 and have them evaluated and properly treated. This is a very hard position to be in, and you'll need support also, from either a therapist or a support group. And while disclosing your intentions regarding suicidality may indeed lead to a hospitalization, this may be the pathway that you need at this time in order to be properly medicated and treated.

One hallmark of depression is that when you're in the depths, it can be very hard to remember that feelings are transitory and you'll not always feel this way. Also, it's the nature of true depression that it's extremely difficult to make yourself do the things that could make you feel better, like going on a short walk or taking a shower. And indeed, one of the reasons you might be depressed is that you're not even *capable* of doing your old strategies for keeping depression at bay, like exercising. You're going to need entirely new coping strategies.

Communication and Emotions

It's really hard to communicate when you're depressed. By definition, you're feeling hopeless about everything; what could there possibly be to talk about? Yet you're both going through a terrible time, and if you don't connect, you may start to diverge onto separate paths and be unable to help one another. If you're the ill partner, try to express how you're feeling to your partner, along with letting them know what you think might be helpful and how they can help. If your partner suggests mental health assistance, try to understand that they may be able to see the situation more clearly than you can right now, and take their advice.

If you're the well partner and feeling really depressed, you may feel like you cannot express this to your partner. After all, they're the sick one; how could you bring them down *even more*? And you don't want them to feel guilty that their illness is making you depressed. Try being honest about how you're feeling, while reassuring your partner that you're responsible for your own feelings and will be getting some outside help to deal with your depression; perhaps by saying something like "I want you to know that I'm feeling depressed. This isn't your responsibility, and I'm working on it, but I just wanted you to know." While in the depression phase, it's important to communicate with one another, but also not to expect your partner to be your sole support during this time.

Shared Activity

There's no question that many activities can play a role in relieving depression. Exercise in particular has been shown to have an antidepressant effect. Yet the reason you're depressed is because your life has fallen apart and exercise may be contraindicated (as it is for many chronic illnesses) or impossible. If you're not the depressed partner, ask your partner what they feel would be possible and feel good that you could do together. Even if it's lying under a blanket on the couch and just holding each other, that counts as a shared activity. With depression, it's tempting to isolate yourself, so doing any shared activity with another person is a step in the right direction. Keep in mind that when you're depressed you will not *want* to do any helpful activity; wanting to do it is not the point. If you know cognitively that it's something that is helpful for depression, and it's possible for you to do it, do it.

Intimacy and Sex

The problem with depression is that you simply have no energy or capacity for pleasure. Many find no pleasure in previously pleasurable activities, and sex and intimacy can fall into this category. You're not motivated to do *anything*, much less engage in sexual activity. I've said that touch is very healing for human beings, yet because isolating oneself is part of the depression package, often we deny ourselves the healing power of our partner's touch. Be clear with one another that you may not have the energy or capacity to engage in intense sexual activity right now, but you don't want to forgo healthy touch. If you're the nondepressed partner, ask your partner what kind of touch they can tolerate that would feel healing to them. If you're depressed together, force yourselves to engage in some kind of touch each day, whether sexual or nonsexual. If you just can't bring yourself to be touched at all, try lying next to each other under weighted blankets, so that you at least have a shared experience of intimacy.

Friends, Family, and Gatekeeping

Most people cannot tolerate depression. The world is so full of toxic positivity—just say your affirmations and feel better!—that you likely don't know what to do with your negative feelings. Friends and family often discount negative feelings and try to talk you into feeling how you "should" be feeling and hoping for all the things you "should" be hopeful for. Obviously this isn't helpful. On the other hand, simply ghosting people or isolating yourself can cause a bigger problem: their trying even *harder* to cheer you up. You may need to be very clear with those around you that you're experiencing hopelessness and depression, and that this is a natural part of the grieving cycle of chronic illness. You can simply be firm: "Depression is a natural part of adjusting to chronic illness, and I don't need you to fix it for me." If you know what would be helpful from your friends and family, let them know explicitly. For example, if you can't get out of bed to do your laundry, ask someone to help you with it. Most people love to feel useful—that's what they're *trying* to accomplish by trying to cheer you up—but you may need to tell them that something else would be more helpful. Many people need to hear that just sitting with you in the despair is helpful. For most people, this feels like they're not doing anything helpful, and it even feels counterproductive. But if it's helpful to you to just have someone witness your despair and sit with you without talking, you may need to actually tell them that, practice in small chunks, and reinforce afterward how helpful that was!

Chronic illness generates a lot of input from other people—your friends and family, the medical community, even social media. When you're depressed, you may need to really limit this, as it can just add to an already intolerable burden. I suggest taking a media fast at least; there's nothing on the internet that won't still be there when you're feeling better. You may also want to postpone your nonurgent medical appointments to a time when you can better advocate for yourself. This is a marathon, not a sprint; it's okay to take breaks.

Let's consider the case in which *both* of you are depressed. Much that I've talked about here requires one partner—who isn't depressed—to step in and help the other partner, who is. But what if you're both severely depressed? You can't really support each other or brainstorm ideas. In this case, it might be useful to "open a gate" for a person outside your relationship to help. Is there someone in your sphere you would trust to check in and encourage the two of you to get help? This person might take care of tasks you need done, make appointments for you, or find you a therapist. While gatekeeping is usually about building a gate so you don't get exposure to too many outside influences, it can also be a way of letting in people who are helpful to you.

Reflection Questions

1. Have you ever experienced depression before, or is this the first time you've had this experience?
2. Do you find yourself withdrawing from your partner and other sources of support? Are there any tiny ways you feel you can connect?
3. What is the smallest healthy step you feel you're capable of taking?

Coping with Depression

This may be the most complex phase, because depression impairs your critical thinking *and* your energy level. Your ability to "work" on your depression may come and go or disappear altogether. Be patient with yourself through this phase. When you do have some energy, ACT has some ideas for coping and dealing with depression.

ACT Skill: The Observing Self

The ACT skill we'll learn here is called the observing self or self-as-context. Confusing names and entirely unnecessary for you to understand, really. What you need to understand is that there are two yous. There's the you who's reading this content and thinking to yourself *What in the world?*, and there's the you who can think about the fact that you're reading. There are the thoughts you're having, and the part of you that can sit back and watch yourself thinking that.

Let's use metaphors. Think about a sky filled with clouds, which are your thoughts and feelings, always moving through—sometimes dark, sometimes light and puffy, but not intrinsically part of the sky itself. The sky itself cannot be damaged by the clouds; they're simply an overlay. The sky is the part of you that is above all the thoughts and feelings. The religious might call it a "soul," or you might think of it as your core essence, or your deep self that is connected to all things. Another metaphor (that you'll recognize from earlier in the book) is leaves on a river—the leaves are just floating past, constantly moving and changing. But the river is more of a constant, not really affected at its core by the leaves coming and going.

It's helpful, when depressed, to understand that depression isn't *you*. *You're* not depressed. You have feelings and emotions of depression. They may be setting in for a long storm, or they may just be passing through. But behind all of that is the real you that can't be damaged by those thoughts or feelings or even your chronic illness symptoms. This isn't to diminish your very strong and real feelings. It's just to say that's not all you are. You're not your feelings. You're not your symptoms.

This might sound too spiritual for you if you don't tend toward spiritual thinking. But it's not really spiritual. You can think of it however you want or need to think of it. The main idea is to see the depression as something that is happening *to* you, just as your symptoms are happening to you, but they are not *you*.

Will thinking this way resolve your depression automatically? I'm sorry, no. Feelings of depression are heavy and pervasive, and you aren't really trying to get rid of them right now. The idea that "what you resist, persists" is true, in that the more you try to get rid of your depression, the more depression tends to set in. What you're trying to do here is get perspective on your depression; that it's temporary, fluid, and not who you *are*. It's simply something that is moving through you like a cloud, and underneath all of those clouds, you're still you.

Since I tend toward depression myself, I cherish the ultimate knowledge from past experience that I won't always feel this way. Depression is a liar, convincing you that nothing will ever and can ever get better. But that's not how feelings work. Scientifically, it's almost impossible for you to feel exactly as you do now forever and always. So even in the depths of feeling awful, I try to remind myself this is a temporary overlay on my life now, but if I do any and all healthy things I'm capable of, I *will* wake up one day and feel different. So far, it's been true every time.

Depression is a stage. You might move through this stage many times, or not at all. You might move through it together as partners or experience it at different times. Like all stages, it will shift and change over time. Feel the stability of the river or sky inside you and know that none of the feelings can hurt you if you allow them to just move through.

Reflection Questions

1. Does knowing there is more to you than what you're experiencing now give you a shift in perspective that seems helpful?
2. What does the kindest, wisest part of you want you to know about what you're going through?

Chapter Summary Points

- Depression often happens when you've tried many remedies that have failed and you still feel terrible.
- Depression can happen at any point, though, and is an entirely normal reaction to having a chronic, incurable condition.
- Suicidal thoughts are somewhat normal, but finding profession help is crucial if this is part of your experience.
- It can be hard to support one another through depression, but communicating about your feelings helps you stay connected.
- Gaining perspective on your depression as separate from your core self can be helpful.
- Get in touch with the you who cannot be touched by external circumstances, and draw strength from the stability of this core self.

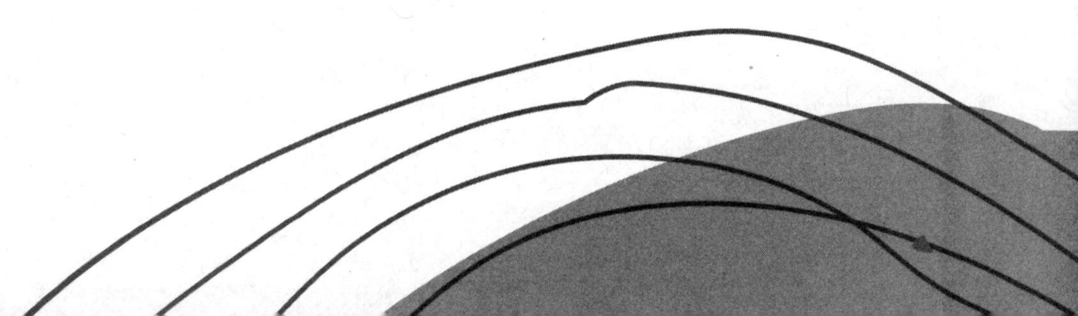

Moving On

Depression is a very difficult phase of chronic illness, and largely unavoidable. No one likes to be depressed, yet it's really hard to do what might help to alleviate your symptoms. Also, if one of you is depressed and not the other, support may be hard to achieve, yet if both of you are depressed, it can be hard to brainstorm ideas for feeling better. In the next chapter we'll look at some practical concerns each of you might have and practice some tools that could move the needle, even just slightly.

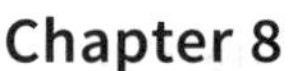

Chapter 8

Tools for the Depression Phase

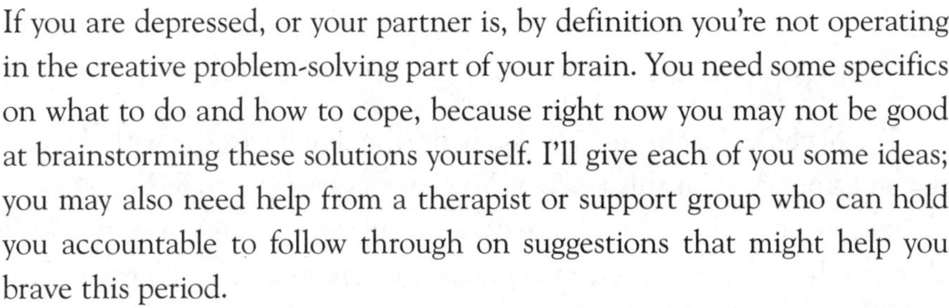

If you are depressed, or your partner is, by definition you're not operating in the creative problem-solving part of your brain. You need some specifics on what to do and how to cope, because right now you may not be good at brainstorming these solutions yourself. I'll give each of you some ideas; you may also need help from a therapist or support group who can hold you accountable to follow through on suggestions that might help you brave this period.

How You May Be Feeling

Most likely, you're both going to experience depression at some point in this process, either at the same time or at different points, and either once or multiple times through the years. Again, depression is entirely normal for *each* of you, although the reasons for your depression may differ. Because you may be depressed for different reasons, you may easily get impatient with one another, or downplay the other person's concerns. Depression, while devastating, isn't *who* you or your partner are at your core. It's a natural experience, and one that will likely ebb and flow. The more empathetic and loving you can be toward one another, the better.

Well Partner

If your partner is the one who's depressed, it can be excruciatingly hard to witness. I'm sure you understand *why* they are depressed; no one wants to be sick without any hope of a cure. But it can be hard to know what to do about it. You instinctively want to make them feel better, but you know by now that just trying to "cheer someone up" doesn't usually work. But you also don't want to get down in the mire with them! It's confusing. If you're the one depressed, you may feel like there's no space for you to feel that. Your partner may be unsympathetic to your depression, because after all, *you're* the one who still has a life and is well! Or they might be sympathetic, but you feel the burden of not wanting to bring them further down when they have enough problems already. So many different dynamics could be at play, I can't possibly cover them all here, but I'll try to give you some ideas.

Sick Partner

I've never had a chronic illness client who didn't struggle with depression at some point on this journey. You have every right to feel depressed; it's entirely normal. You used to have a life, plans, dreams—now that's all changed. If you've experienced depression before, maybe you have a strategy for getting through these feelings, but maybe it's entirely new for you. Depression's hallmarks include isolation and lack of energy, which is problematic because many helpful healing actions require energy and other people. But all you want to do is pull the covers over your head and make everyone and everything just *go away*. You might even be having scary thoughts about suicide, which you've never had before. If you're overwhelmed by these thoughts or preoccupied with making plans in that direction, *please* tell your partner and seek professional help.

On the other hand, your partner may be the one who's depressed right now. This might feel outrageous to you. They can still go paddleboarding! They can still work! They can still go to the gym! How *dare* they be depressed when you're the one whose life has been ruined by illness! Do your best to muster some compassion for how this situation has impacted your partner as well. They were also just going along in their life when this happened; and because you're a team, what happens to you affects them. I get that you're dealing with a physical illness that saps your energy and takes a lot of your time, so I'm not asking you to be the sole support of your partner while they are depressed. But if you can at least be empathetic, that will help.

Communication and Emotions

As you likely know, a depressed person is likely to either struggle to communicate or stop altogether. If you're both working on this issue, try to design a cadence and way of communicating that works for both of you. Since communication isn't likely to come naturally here, try "Let's check in once a day just for ten minutes so we can share how we are feeling." An established appointment is less likely to fall by the wayside. When you convene, you both should have a chance to explain how you're feeling and suggest any practical actions that could be helpful. If either of you is having suicidal thoughts, try to develop a plan for addressing this. Therapists are generally trained to ask directly, "Are you feeling suicidal today?" and then, if the answer is yes, "Do you have any plan for acting on these thoughts?" I know this is a scary conversation to have, but obviously a very important one. If you can commit to being honest with one another, you can make agreements, such as empathizing with these naturally occurring thoughts, but also committing to some type of action if the thoughts become more than just thoughts. If you don't feel that you can support each other in this way (which is natural), intentionally designate some other trusted person to track these thoughts and behaviors so somebody is checking in and monitoring for danger.

Well Partner

If you're the depressed one, your feelings are entirely valid. You're still well physically, but your life has been turned upside down too, and you're allowed to have feelings about it. While many of us got together with our partners so that they could be our person, your partner might not be the best one to support you right now. They're dealing with a lot themself, and you don't want them to feel guilty or upset that they're also "ruining" your life. However, it's important to be honest about what you're feeling so you don't give mixed messages. Tell your partner that you're experiencing depression; reassure them that your feelings are your responsibility, and let them know what you'll be doing for support.

If your partner is the one who is depressed, try not to be frustrated with them. It's hard to imagine having to deal with an illness that'll never abate, so depression is a completely normal reaction, and the more that you can help normalize it for your partner, the better. If your partner isn't sharing their depression with you, you may need to tell them you notice they are depressed and that this is normal; then ask them directly what you can do to support them. It's a very loving act to say something like "It seems to me that you're depressed. I think that's normal for what you're going through. Is there something specific I can be doing to help you through this?"

Sick Partner

When people are depressed, usually the last thing they want to do is talk about it. Most people with depression tend to withdraw from their friends and activities and isolate in their home or room. When things feel hopeless, what's there to even say? Resisting your depression isn't going to help you make any progress, but sharing what you're feeling might help lighten the load. It's hard when the last thing you want to do is communicate, but you can keep it brief. Saying something like "I feel so depressed about where I'm at. I know it won't last forever, but can I just get a hug?" at least lets your partner in on your process. They deserve to know how you're feeling and what would be helpful to you. Try to include your partner in your healing process when possible, and accept their influence if they are encouraging you to do things known to be helpful.

If your partner is the depressed one, try to communicate that their feelings are valid and you understand why this situation would create depression for them. If you don't feel capable of helping them, let them know that while you empathize, you can't be their sole support. Encourage them to get some outside support—therapy, a support group, or a wise friend who might give good counsel. The main thing is to communicate with one another and validate how normal feelings of depression can be.

EXERCISE: Daily Check-In

Open communication is the key in this phase of chronic illness. Chronic illness *is depressing*. But especially if only one of you is depressed, you can quickly lose contact with one another if you let isolation rule the day. Set aside a reasonably doable time each day to check in; I suggest ten minutes, but find out what works for you. Thinking about the different categories, decide what you might need to check in about each day. For example, sex might be no problem for you, but you need to check on suicidality every day. Or maybe friends and family all understand, but you need to check in about intimate connection. Commit yourselves to brief daily check-ins on these topics, and try to discover one practical, helpful thing your partner could do for you. It's easy to become overwhelmed when depressed, so giving just one task to your partner is much easier than discussing your entire relationship.

EXERCISE: Communicate and Offer Help

If your partner is depressed, try to communicate clearly with them. Let them know you understand and know that depression is entirely normal and there's nothing wrong with the feelings they're having. Ask what kind of help you can give, whether that's finding a therapist, making appointments, or taking on extra tasks. Encourage them to engage in doable activities that might move the needle even a bit. Let them know what kind of outside support *you* will be getting while they are unable to do this for you.

Shared Activity

Shared activity is really tough during this phase, because it's kind of a double whammy. Not only are your shared activities limited by the sick partner's physical symptoms, but now you're also dealing with symptoms of depression. While the physical symptoms may be permanent and unrelenting, depression should be a temporary setback. The key is to openly discuss what feels possible for both parties, realizing you may have to think in a very scaled-back way. Just watching a funny show together or eating dinner together counts. When shared activities aren't possible, it may be a shared activity just to talk about and plan future activities that you can't do now but may be able to at some point. Ask your partner to have a "let's dream about something in the future" conversation.

Well Partner

If your partner is depressed, they'll likely not want to do anything; that's the nature of depression. It's not helpful to try to drag your partner out of bed to go for a walk or movie, or try to do the things that you normally do. However, it's okay to challenge your partner to do small things that might take them in a healing direction. So, for example, if you normally go for a short evening walk, ask them if they'd just come sit on the porch with you for ten minutes to get some evening air. Reassure them that they don't have to talk or expend any additional energy. Start with the smallest steps that might be doable.

If you're the depressed partner, similarly try to push yourself to do small things that might make a difference. If you'll do these things with your partner, try to be clear about what you are and aren't capable of. If you can sit on the porch but don't feel capable of a conversation, just say so. Again, it's important to understand that you don't have to *want* to do something, or feel like doing something, in order to do it. If you know cognitively it would be good for you, try to make the effort.

Sick Partner

Probably activities you used to share have already been curtailed by your physical limitations. So you may already not be doing much with your partner, and I'd like to make the argument that this might be contributing to your (or your partner's) depression. If you didn't want to do shared activities with a person, you wouldn't choose that person as a friend. Now here you are—*the* person that you each chose as *your* person—and not doing anything together. Not only do you have physical limitations, but one of you is depressed and even *more* likely to not want to do anything.

There are many sedentary activities that don't require a lot of energy and attention; I encourage you to brainstorm these options. Even if you're just snuggled up and touching while you're each reading a book, I'll take it.

EXERCISE: Provide Support and Ideas for Your Partner

If your partner is depressed, cultivate compassion and empathy for their experience. Communicate with them clearly. Sit down with them to acknowledge that you notice their depression, to let them know how you're capable of helping (if you are), and suggest outside support for them. Invite them to keep you updated on their feelings and emotions as they move through. It's hard to be creative when depressed, so ask your partner to brainstorm with you the smallest activities they think they can manage—sitting in the backyard, taking a bath, or just cuddling.

Intimacy and Sex

As we've discussed in other chapters, communication in any relationship is hard, and talking about sex is exponentially *more* difficult. This may be a rough topic for you already, if the physical symptoms have made your old rhythms and patterns impossible. But depression will certainly compound this, because depression by its nature isn't interested in pleasurable activities. I'd like you both to acknowledge, if you can, that different forms of intimacy are an important part of a romantic relationship. If you were single and you met someone you had no physical interest in, you wouldn't put them in the relationship bucket—you'd put them in the friendship bucket. It's really the one thing that decidedly separates this relationship from all other relationships that you might pursue. So what do you do when that part of your relationship breaks down? If you can both agree that this is vital, that's helpful, because then you can brainstorm creative ways to maintain this connection even within the limited context in which you're now living. Sex might not be possible, or even desired, if you're in a depressive phase. What else can you do to connect that feels good? Does taking a bath together appeal? Sharing a jacuzzi? Getting a couples' massage? Could you just snuggle up together without anything more? Try to brainstorm ideas that don't take much energy but could provide you with connection and healing energy.

Well Partner

Sex generally requires energy, and depressed people often lack this type of liveliness. It's both respectful and okay for couples to decide that sex is off the table for a short period while one of them is dealing with deep depression. Remember, intimacy and sex are two different things, and touch is healing. Try to be open about whether either of you has the energy for sex, and if not, whether you can incorporate any calm touch.

Also, one or both of you may be depressed *because* of sex, especially if sex isn't possible because of your partner's illness. Again, this is valid and understandable if sex has disappeared from your life since this illness began. It helps to keep the communication open and be creative about touch and intimacy. Tell your partner, "I'm sad that we've lost our sexual connection right now—and it seems like you are too, But we can still connect. Let's think of some ways we can touch and be sensual now."

Sick Partner

Many people do not want to have sex when they are depressed. One symptom of depression is not being interested in activities that are normally pleasurable, and one of the main points of sex is giving and receiving pleasure—so it makes sense that it wouldn't appeal when depression sets in. As I've said so many times, sex and intimacy aren't the same thing. Touch is healing for almost everyone. Communicate clearly during this time, whether it's you or your partner who is depressed. Discuss whether there are any options for intimacy that seem doable for you, such as lying on the couch just snuggling. You may not *feel* like doing this right now, but try to commit to the behavior even if the feelings don't come along. Everything you do in this regard is a tiny step in the right direction, but it may take some time for your feelings to change.

EXERCISE: Notice Pleasure

Since an absence of pleasure is a symptom of depression, it makes sex and intimacy difficult. Sit down together and brainstorm tiny activities that you know have brought you pleasure in the past. This might be holding hands, getting a foot rub, snuggling on the couch, or breathing together. Practice self-as-context by noticing that a part of you is depressed, while at the same time, there's a part of you that can still feel the sensations of this activity. Try to practice the perspective that the depression is a part of you but can't diminish your ability to feel sensual sensation.

Friends, Family, and Gatekeeping

The world can be overwhelming to a depressed person. And if you're not both depressed, the nondepressed partner might be wanting all kinds of outside support, while that support is feeling smothering to the depressed partner. Talk together about what kind of outside support is helpful to each of you at this time—it doesn't have to be the same, as long as you can support one another in getting your needs met. Try to decide if there are people or outside influences (like doctors' offices and social media) it would be helpful for you to disconnect from temporarily. If so, come up with a united plan to do this together. If one person needs outside support and the other doesn't, allow for that activity to support that partner. In depression specifically, there may be times you'll need to encourage the depressed partner to engage with others even when they don't want to. This can feel insulting, but try to remember that sometimes the nondepressed partner can see what you need better than you can see it yourself. Make these interactions brief and low-energy initially. For example, you might say to a friend "I'm feeling depressed and I'm not up for much, but maybe we could FaceTime just for five minutes?"

If your partner is the depressed one, try not to jump on the bandwagon with friends and family in terms of cheering them up. In general, people don't like to be around depressed people and don't understand depression, so you might need to educate your family and friends that depression is a normal part of this process, and help them to understand what's helpful. Also, be careful of getting extensive support from people in your circle by talking to them about things that you should be talking about with your partner or a professional. It can be very easy to become emotionally drawn to another person when your partner is "offline" with depression.

Well Partner

If you're the depressed partner, you may need to ask your partner to do some gatekeeping for you. But because your partner is physically ill, they may not be capable of taking on this role. Try to see if there's someone who can field calls, return calls, and so forth while you have some space to heal. If it's your partner who's depressed, you can offer to do these are things for them if it's helpful—or just ask them how you can help intervene to protect them from the outside world.

Sick Partner

If it's your partner who's depressed, and especially if you're outraged about that, you might be tempted to make others outraged as well. After all, you're the victim here! Getting people to join in on your "side" might feel validating, but it's not good for your relationship overall. If you can communicate to others that your partner is depressed and that's normal, your partner will likely experience this as very supportive. You might also ask specifically for certain friends or family to regularly connect with your partner so they can get the support they need.

On the other hand, if you're the one who's depressed, you might need to figure out which of your friends and family might be helpful to you right now, and specifically what they could do that would be helpful. You can also ask your partner to relay this information if you just don't feel capable of doing it.

EXERCISE: Get Perspective

If you're depressed, try to get some perspective on who you are versus the depression that is happening *to* you. Just like the sky with clouds moving through, the sky itself is untouched by whatever storm is raging. Somewhere underneath all of this depression and all of your symptoms is the real you. Who is that person? If you're inclined toward creativity, perhaps you can draw a portrait of the you who observes all of this happening to you. Who is that person? It can help to externalize your symptoms and your depression as if they are characters on the stage of your life—but you're the actual stage. Giving your symptoms or depression names or faces that are separate from you can sometimes help give you a little space to still exist despite all the dark clouds.

EXERCISE: Creative Values Project

Look back at the values that you've created as a team. (If you're reading this book out of order and haven't created your values yet, you may need to flip to that chapter and do that exercise first.) Use one of the metaphors I've described to think about the situation you're in now. For example, if you've defined your values together, those values are the "sky" of your relationship. That is the stable, solid part that exists regardless of whatever outside circumstances or feelings might be happening. Then talk about the things that are happening as if they are clouds just moving past the stable sky. If you're artistic, you may even create a visual to remind you that what's happening to you as a couple is separate from who you really are. For example, let's say you create a felt backboard that represents the sky. You could create all kinds of small felt pieces that represent different experiences—depression, pain, fatigue, and so on. You and your partner could decorate the sky each day as a visual representation of the outside influences you're personally experiencing on any given day—and be reminded that the sky is still there behind all of the distress.

Moving On

I'm so sorry that you've needed to read these last two chapters, because no one wants to have to experience deep depression. Depression can be pervasive and sometimes dangerous, so I encourage you to contact a professional if the suggestions in this chapter don't seem to be enough to help you through this phase. Be gentle with each other, and put the focus on communication.

Next, we are going to talk about testing, and coming up with concrete, workable plans for the future.

Chapter 9

Testing and Acceptance

What You Will Learn in This Chapter:

- Testing and acceptance is a stage, not a permanent state.
- As things change, you may reach this stage and also move out of this stage from time to time.
- Testing out options has a more stable and calm feel than bargaining.
- Acceptance does *not* mean that this is okay or that you're giving up.
- Committed actions are actions in line with your values.
- You may have to brainstorm new goals that align with your values, and then commit to moving toward these new goals.
- You can behave according to your committed action no matter how you're feeling emotionally.

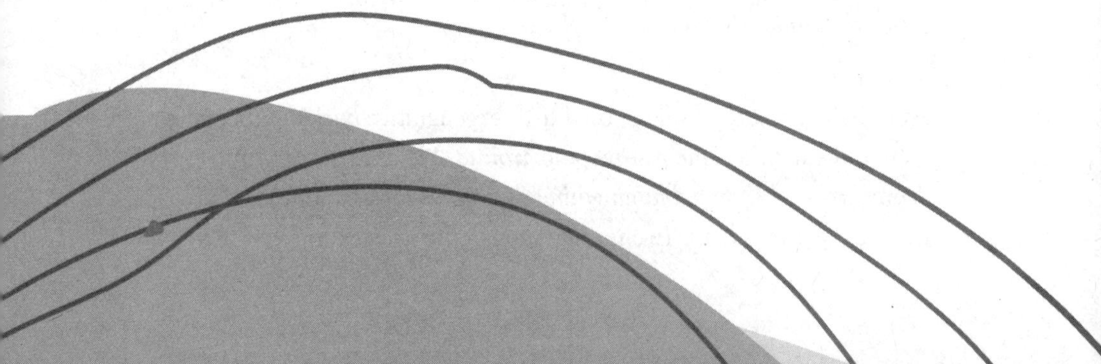

The couples we met in the bargaining chapter can demonstrate now how things look different in testing and acceptance.

It seems like Juanita has tried every intervention on the planet for fibromyalgia. Many didn't work, and some even made her feel sicker. She spent about a year in deep despair, wondering if her life would ever be worth living again. Slowly, though, something came back alive for Juanita. She and Tim started communicating more about what was going on, and she learned something new: Tim could actually be empathetic. Juanita thought about her life before fibromyalgia, coaching sports for kids. One of her life values is inspiring the next generation. So Juanita found a few things that worked for her pain most of the time, and she developed a new online program for at-risk kids that she can do even when she's not feeling well. Juanita is still sick, and she may always be. But she loves the new life she's built and feels proud of herself for working within her boundaries.

It took Tim a long time to come around. He was so angry with all the money being spent on miracle cures and the ups and downs that Juanita was going through; meanwhile, it seemed like his *needs were never considered. But at a certain point, Tim realized that his anger and way of dealing with this situation wasn't helping at all. He knows he can't just keep doing the same things, so he's decided to try empathy and more communication. One of Tim's life values is kindness and understanding, and he came to realize he wasn't doing this for Juanita. And kind of a miracle happened—once he was more empathetic and supportive of Juanita, she became more open to meeting his needs. It's not always the way he wants it; they don't work out together anymore, and they don't have sex as much as he'd like. But they spend a lot of time snuggling and talking, and Tim feels closer to Juanita than ever.*

After Mohammad was diagnosed with degenerative back disease, he spent quite a bit of time just moping around. He went straight into depression and shame, blaming himself and his lack of faith for the way his life turned out. Eventually, though, he decided to go back to the mosque and at least wrestle with Allah over what had become of him. In this process, he met with the imam of his mosque, and the imam encouraged him to worship, but also to take advantage of available treatments. He noted that Islam's value system gives utmost priority to good health. Because Mohammad shares this value, he committed to pursuing any available treatments. While there is no cure for Mohammad's disease, he now lives a much more comfortable life and feels a dedication toward living in the best health he can achieve.

Asmaa couldn't be happier that Mohammad finally yielded to the good counsel of the imam and pursued treatment. She didn't know how to reach Mohammad during his dark period and resented how he didn't accept her influence in terms of what they should do. Because she shares his faith, she was able to join with him in defining their life values and figuring out helpful ways to pursue them. Now Asmaa and Mohammad are aligned in their values and faith, so they're able to really work as a team.

The Lay of the Land

I decided to revisit the couples from the bargaining chapter (chapter 5) as an example of how this process can proceed to some sort of resolution. Now, testing and acceptance are still phases. You may land here and find some peace from time to time; then something changes, and you have to rework the process. This doesn't equal failure, but shows that as things change—science, your symptoms, your life circumstances—new feelings and challenges may come up, and the peacefulness you may have temporarily found may be shattered. It's okay. Just go back to some of the earlier chapters and revisit the tools you learned there. Just like any other feeling phase, testing and acceptance aren't permanent states.

Testing is kind of at the opposite end of the spectrum from bargaining. There's a frenzied quality to bargaining, and it's driven by an "if only" motivation. In bargaining, you find yourself flitting from idea to idea, treatment to treatment, in pursuit of something that might help. But in testing, you have a more methodical approach. You've done your experiments; you've found a few things that help a little some of the time. You may have found a cluster of things that together create a more manageable life. In the testing mode, you can prioritize what works for you and what doesn't and what kind of intervals these treatments need; you're managing the costs of treatment responsibly. You're aligned with your partner in how you each approach these options, and you've found some kind of agreement, even if you don't feel exactly the same.

When you're living in the period of testing, you may still have false starts, periods of "failure." But you see this as part of the process and are not devastated by it. This leads you to a form of acceptance. I emphasize: Acceptance does *not* mean you think what has happened to you is okay. It does *not* mean you've given up. It simply means that you're clear about the reality of the situation and not tossed about by every emotion and piece of information that comes your way.

Here are some examples of acceptance in the memoirs I have previously mentioned:

> What does it mean for a chronically ill patient to heal? In some cases, it may mean a remission of disease. But in others, it means the patient is now able to manage the illness with some degree of integrity…it's not being cured necessarily, but feeling whole. (O'Rourke 2023)

> But the most basic blessing woven into the burden of a chronic illness has been the opportunity to keep going on, to remain there as a father and a husband even in a diminished state…the chance to keep going also includes the chance to keep fighting, keep searching for answers, to keep hoping for a cure. (Douthat 2021)

> The fostering, the nourishment, the tending to myself, the commitment to daily ritual, the trusting of my own feelings and intuition, the emphasis on connection, the willingness to change, and the acceptance and surrender to the dark aspects of myself…if you've been crushed, and crushed and then crushed again, remember…the Book of the Dead is also the book of life. (Ramey 2020)

What do you notice about these quotes? These aren't people who have given up. They're people who continue to fight, day after day—for treatments, for information, for a cure. But they're also people who've defined what their values are, what they're actually living for, and how they want to proceed with integrity and intention.

You don't ever have to like what has happened to you. But I'd like you to never give up. And you might hit this sweet spot from time to time where—both individually and as a team—you can clearly and thoughtfully decide on a way forward and live your life with intention while you're doing that. No state is permanent, so if you're approaching or have achieved this state, try to enjoy it.

Communication and Emotions

As with many of these stages, communication is critical if you're going to reach this one together. If you're the sick partner, you may have tried a zillion things and then plunged into depression, and it's helpful for the well partner to know that you're emerging from this dark place with some semblance of a plan. The well partner might think this is a regression back into the frenzied period of bargaining, and it's important to let them know that this is different. If you haven't communicated your values to your partner, you may need to help them understand what you've discovered about your values, and how that influences the way you'd like to live going forward. Then be open to their feedback about your plan and how your plan will affect their life. They may have some different ideas about your plan, based on how it affects them, and it's fair to consider this and potentially alter that plan.

If you're the well partner, you also might be emerging from periods of anger or despair, when it seemed like you'd never have a life worth living again, at least if you stay in this relationship. In the period of testing and acceptance, you may have found some things that work for you to live this life with integrity, and you need to explain to your partner what that looks like. For example, you may have realized that a quarterly retreat with the Well Spouse organization (see Resources) keeps you feeling recharged and flush with community support. Going to these retreats has you feeling in touch with your values of caring for your partner, but also gives you much-needed camaraderie. Your partner doesn't love to be left alone while you're off socializing, but it's a solution you can both live with.

Shared Activity

Throughout the book, we've talked about how shared activity takes a hit when one of you gets sick and is too fatigued or down to participate. The stage of testing and acceptance means that you've talked about and agreed to an experimentation process that honors where both of you are. For example, let's say you used to play tennis together. Now one of you can't do that, but the other one joins a Saturday morning league, and when the sick partner feels up to it, they go and watch. Because they often go and cheer on the well partner, it feels like something you're still doing together. You can talk together about today's game and upcoming tournaments, and it's still something you have in common.

Or let's say that you used to travel extensively and now the sick partner can't do that. You decide to join the "armchair traveler" group at the library and "visit" all kinds of places together. It's not what you had planned for your lives, but it's something that you can do together and enjoy. Sometimes you might test out options that don't work. You used to paddleboard together, and now the sick partner can't stand for that long. So you get a kayak for the sick partner to sit in and paddle alongside. Unfortunately, it turns out the fatigue of your partner's illness doesn't allow for this kind of exertion. In the testing phase, the attitude is "That didn't work, but it was worth a try." You can accept that not all experiments will be successful.

Intimacy and Sex

Most partners go through a long period of anger and resentment about the change in sexual behavior. That makes sense, because in monogamous relationships, this is a need you can't satisfy elsewhere. In the testing phase, you've begun to realize that you're not going to get back to exciting sex three times a week, like before you got sick. But you also realize now that intimacy is more than just sex, and you're committed to being as physically intimate as possible. If sex is possible, you've come up with a frequency schedule that is doable for both partners and options for when it isn't, like cuddling or self-stimulation. You actually touch a lot more than you ever did before when you just went straight to intercourse. Now you snuggle in bed reading, you hold hands on the couch when you're watching TV, and you give each other sweet massages when you have the energy to do so. You're both committed to making sure the other person knows that they are desired and loved in a physical way.

In some situations, to achieve this end, you may need to discuss whether an open relationship or other form of ethical nonmonogamy is an option for you. This option isn't for everyone, and if you have a strong negative reaction to it right off the bat, it might not be for you. But if you're the sick partner and you have a strong negative reaction, you may want to explore how your partner feels about it. In years past, this option wasn't even discussed as a viable option, but these days many people are pursuing polyamorous or open relationships with success. I suggest reading books such as *Polywise* and *Polysecure* by Jessica Fern, or receiving some professional assistance as you design this new possibility.

Friends, Family, and Gatekeeping

It takes some time and experimentation to get your family and friends on board. You've likely had many frustrating experiences and missteps by the time you get to this phase in the process. You might have invited ideas and input and then become overwhelmed by it. Maybe you told your families something you thought was private, and they blasted it out on Facebook before you were ready. Maybe people haven't been helpful, or maybe they've been so overly helpful that you feel smothered. Maybe you've completely isolated yourself from people, or maybe you've raged on people when you thought they were inconsiderate.

Now you're able to look at the bigger picture and see times when people have been helpful and times when they haven't. In the testing and acceptance phase, you're able to clearly communicate with other people—without passive aggressiveness—what's been helpful for you and what hasn't. You're able to ask directly for the things that are helpful and set clear boundaries when they're not.

Similarly to friends and family issues, there've been times when you've been overwhelmed and irate at the medical system. There's no question that the medical system we have (at least in the United States) isn't designed to be useful or comfortable for those of us with chronic illness. So in other phases, you might be consumed with anger or despair over the way you've been treated. In this phase, you and your partner have been able to really create a dance that works in terms of how you communicate with doctors, how and at what pacing you go to appointments, whether you both go, and who communicates with your team of doctors.

Not only medically, but with all input (including social media), you've figured out who is good at setting the boundaries and come up with a system for doing that. You still don't *like* that you've to set so many boundaries, but you know how to do it, and you're consistent at following through.

Reflection Questions

1. Have you found any behaviors or solutions to your illness that seem to consistently work for you to feel better?
2. What kinds of communication or teamwork have helped in your partnership together?
3. Have you experienced any moments, no matter how brief, of acceptance about the reality of your situation?

Coping in Testing and Acceptance

This phase feels pretty good (compared with those that came before), and there's less urgent need for coping skills. But it takes certain skills to reach the testing and acceptance phase and hopefully sustain you in this phase as long as possible. You'll want to be familiar with the skills ACT has to offer, so you can reach this phase and savor being there.

ACT Skill: Committed Behavior and Acceptance

So, what are the skills needed to make all this happen? In ACT, the skills are committed action and acceptance. Although I've said before that you can read these chapters in any order, you actually do need to have defined your values in order to figure out your committed actions. So if you haven't developed or become clear on your values yet, you'll need to do that now before you can design your committed action.

Committed action means "taking larger and larger patterns of effective action, guided and motivated by values" (Harris 2017, p. 208). One problem with chronic illness is that often your goals aren't compatible with your limitations. In some of the other phases, your feelings have been whipped around by what you're no longer able to do, and you've been angry or depressed about that. But now you can recognize that you're in a reality gap—you have desired goals and outcomes, but the reality is that you aren't going to be able to achieve what you could've achieved before this happened. Reality gaps are painful, and that's why you've likely cycled through some of the other phases before landing here.

So how do you come up with committed actions when your previous goals can't be met? Russ Harris gives us a template in his great book *ACT Made Simple*:

1. First, validate the pain arising from the reality gap.
2. Respond to that pain with acceptance and cognitive defusion.
3. Find the values that are underlying the goals that you had before.
4. Set new goals based on those underlying values. (2017, p. 216)

You can see how this is a much more intentional process than the frenzied activities that happen during the bargaining phase. Here, you intentionally connect with your values to try to figure out the best course of action. Knowing your values helps you to commit to actions that line up with what gives your life meaning, and saves you from pursuing things that may offer empty promises but don't line up with who you really are.

As you're coming up with your list of committed actions, remember that this list may change as new treatments or new symptoms arise. You may have to go through this four-step process many times in your life. One of the beautiful things about committed action is that once you commit to a course of action, you can follow those action steps regardless of what you're feeling. Let's look at an example.

> *Jules was an artist before she got Lyme disease; she was always doing interesting art using welding and metal working. It was demanding physical work, and the sculptures she made were beautiful and stunning. Then came her diagnosis.*
>
> *When Jules gets to a workable point in her disease, she starts longing to get out to her metal shop again. But Jules has a reality gap. There's just no way that Jules is going to have the energy to do that kind of work that she used to do. So Jules takes a look at her values. When Jules looks over the long list of values at newharbinger.com/56081, she chooses "Beauty: to appreciate, create, nurture or cultivate beauty in myself, others, the environment."*
>
> *So Jules needs to set some new goals based on her chosen values. Last week, Jules saw a project that's going to be happening in her local hometown. A group of local knitters is going to be knitting "tree huggers," knitted items that go around all of the trees downtown. Jules is just learning how to knit, but she's got some cool ideas for this project that she really thinks will lend beauty to the downtown landscape. Knitting isn't Jules's first choice for an art activity; she accepts and acknowledges this. But knitting is something she can do, and as long as she stays in touch with the fact that it lines up with her values, it feels like she is still honoring who she wants to be in life.*

Acceptance is kind of like forgiveness, in my opinion. It's not a moment in time. It's not like you reach acceptance and then you're done, that's it, nothing more to do. It's more like you find a place of acceptance and then commit to the *process* of acceptance, which will be easier on some days than on others. But every day when you wake up, you can acknowledge the reality of your situation, connect with your values, and then behave in the ways that are actually possible for you in order to live out those values. Is it the life you wanted? No, no it's not. But it's the life you have, and you're doing everything you can do today to make that life meaningful for yourself and those around you.

Reflection Questions

1. Can you identify any values you have where you might need to work on new goals?
2. How do you feel about the word "acceptance"? Do you have any strong feelings about the possibility of enjoying this feeling, even briefly?

Chapter Summary Points

- Testing means coming up with an intentional list of things to try or things to do that line up with your values.
- Acceptance is merely accepting the reality of how things are today; it doesn't mean that you like it or think what has happened to you is okay.
- Committed actions are goals or ways of behaving that line up with your value system.
- Once you commit to certain actions, you can usually do these things no matter how you're feeling, and it helps life to feel more stable.
- You'll need new goals, since some of your old goals will be unattainable, but the new goals should still line up with your values.

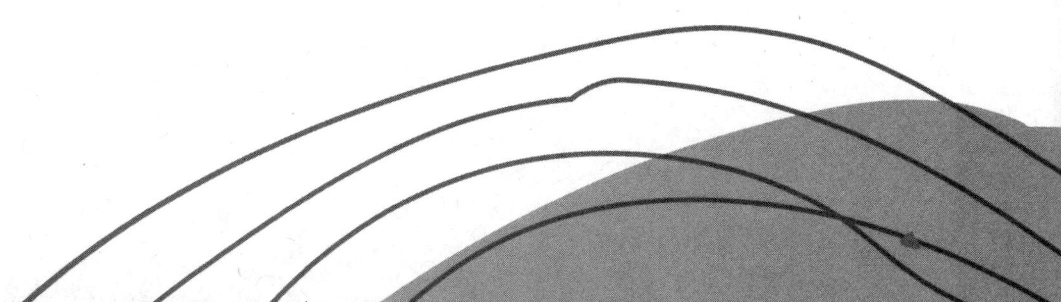

Moving On

This phase can feel a lot better than the other phases we have discussed, more grounded and serene. Remember that this also is just a phase—enjoy it, but don't expect it to last forever! In the next chapter, I'll give you some ideas for moving through this phase as individuals and as partners.

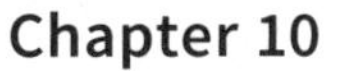

Tools for Testing and Acceptance

The testing and acceptance phase can feel pretty good, like you've arrived someplace. However, you two may not arrive here together. Partners in a chronic illness situation do not always go through the stages together or at the same pace. It can be frustrating to arrive in the testing and acceptance phase and have your partner still angry or depressed. Try to remember that this is just a stage, and you'll also be in darker stages from time to time. I want you to enjoy this period of calm, but you may need a little guidance for what this stage looks like in reality.

How You May Be Feeling

I hope there are at least *some* periods of time that you can spend as a couple in which you're both calm and grounded in the testing and acceptance phase. If that's happening, please enjoy this moment together, where you've found a spot that works for you together and you feel like you've reached a place where life is working for you again. Remind yourselves that this place might not last forever; that's not failure, and you haven't done anything wrong. It's just the nature of the ups and downs of chronic illness that this cannot be a permanent state. But acknowledge to one another how hard you've each worked to get here, and commit to enjoying this phase together as a team.

Well Partner

In the stage of testing and acceptance, you may actually face a few challenges, even though this stage feels good. First, your partner may not be here yet. You may feel adjusted to this new reality (after all, you've got more energy to spend on coping), but your partner is still back in some other stage, and that may feel frustrating to you. Or you may be just now catching up to your partner, who's already here. It's common to not be in the same stage together, and that's okay.

Sick Partner

If you've arrived at the testing and acceptance phase, I want to say I'm proud of you for doing some very hard work to arrive here. You've weathered a huge storm in your life, probably cycled through a lot of uncomfortable stages, and somehow have identified values to get you here, where things feel a bit more manageable. You might feel huge relief that you feel calm and focused, trying new things and finding a blend that works for you in your life. You're not feeling scattered or frantic, but calm and focused as you design your way of life.

However, your partner may not have arrived at this phase with you. If so, you might be struggling to stay grounded if your partner is still depressed or angry, and you might feel guilty for feeling okay when they're still struggling so much. Or you might even feel resentful—*you're* the one with the chronic illness, and if you can accept it, why can't they? Try to remember that even though you're the sick partner, your partner's life has been turned upside down in many ways just as yours has, and they have as much right to work through the process and struggle as you do.

Communication and Emotions

Talk together about what kinds of testing you've done, both individually and together, and what conclusions you've come to. This might seem obvious, but there may be things your partner still does not know regarding your thinking about why things work for you right now or align with your stated values. When you want to test out something new, talk with your partner and explain how and why this aligns with your values and what the testing process may look like. For example, you could say something like "I'd like to test out coming to watch you play tennis on Saturdays. This aligns with my values of being supportive and also getting some fresh air to be healthier. Can we try this out for a few weeks and see how it goes?" In this way, you're keeping each other in the loop about why you're trying things out; then you're following up to see how it's working for each person.

Well Partner

As with all other stages, communication is key. If you're in the testing and acceptance stage, your partner may see this as somewhat of a betrayal, like you've given up on ever figuring out better options for them. Of course this isn't the case, but without communication, your partner won't understand where you're coming from. Try to explain to your partner that you're still there for them emotionally in whatever stage they find themself, and you're available to hear what they are going through. You can say "I don't think we are at the same stage of coping with this illness, and that's okay. I'm feeling like I've figured some things out, but it's okay if you're not there yet." Also explain that you've aligned your values with behaviors that work for you and that you're temporarily resting in a state of acceptance about how things are right now. If your partner is the one in testing and acceptance and you're not, you may feel like your partner is just fine with something that still feels unacceptable to you. Understand that it's a good thing to be able to rest in testing and acceptance for periods, and communicate that you're still working through these changes yourself.

Sick Partner

If you're in the testing and acceptance phase and your partner isn't, this might be a good opportunity to share with them how you got here. If you're here because you've identified your values and are committed to living them even though this illness is in the way, they might benefit from hearing how you achieved that. They may also need to know that you're still committed to learning more about your illness, pursuing new information as it becomes available, and making sure you're following medical advice. If they don't understand the idea of acceptance, perhaps you can explain that your feeling this way means not that you've given up, but that you've accepted that this is your reality for now. Try saying "Sometimes I reach a place where I feel like I can just take a little break from striving so hard for things to be different. I'm just taking a little break; it doesn't mean I've given up trying."

On the other hand, if your partner is in testing and acceptance and you're not there yet, try to appreciate that they've found a grounded place, even if you're a little bit jealous that they've achieved this. Their being grounded and calm does *not* mean that they do not understand your pain, or that they're no longer rooting for you. It only means that they've found some tools that work for them right now, and this may change over time, as it will for you.

EXERCISE: Communicate About Testing

If you and your partner are in this phase together, set aside some time weekly to talk about the things you're testing that are working for you. Check in and see how your conclusions feel for your partner and not just you. Do you both feel the same? If not, can you test some further ideas that might work better for both of you? At the conclusion of each conversation, acknowledge how nice it is to accept reality, even if it's just a temporary phase, and allow yourselves to enjoy it even if it doesn't last forever.

EXERCISE: Gratitude Conversations

Gratitude is great, and there is a lot of science backing up its value. But I think we have to be careful about the potential for toxic positivity. For this reason, I don't suggest gratitude journals for times of anger and/or depression in this context, because it may feel like you're gaslighting yourself, telling yourself that you "should" be feeling grateful. However, if you've temporarily landed in the testing and acceptance phase, it might be a good time to keep a gratitude journal or have a daily gratitude conversation as a couple. You've worked very hard to get here and find ways of being that work for you under these very unfair circumstances. While you're here, it might help and feel good to keep track of the things you're grateful for and your gratitude for the things you've come up with that make your life worth living now. This can be very powerful to do together daily as a team.

Shared Activity

If you're both in this stage, you've likely found activities that work for each of you individually for support, modified activities you can do together as partners, and a division of labor that works and feels at least somewhat fair. Right now you're both feeling like these things align with your values and meet your individual and collective needs. Remember that this isn't a stable state; interests and energy levels change, flare-ups can disturb this calm interlude. Enjoy these activities and time shared together, and communicate as things change. Check in after activities and ask "How was that for you? Does this work in an ongoing way as a way for us to spend time together?" Remind each other that you're committed to sharing time and energy together, but how that looks may change and develop over time.

Well Partner

I hope the two of you have worked through your values, shed the shared activities you used to do that didn't work for you, and brought in new activities that feel much better. If you're in the testing and acceptance phase and your partner isn't, it might be because you've filled your time with activities that fill up your bucket but don't necessarily include your partner. Don't forget that true balance includes at least some activities that you can do together that feel good. If your partner is the one in this phase and you're not, they might feel just fine about the reduced activities between the two of you, while you're still longing for more. Part of testing is trying out new things that align with your values, and you may need to collaborate here so that you both feel good with your level of shared activity.

Sick Partner

Testing in terms of shared activity means that you're now realistic about what is possible for you, and you have an action plan for what kind of energetic expenses you can afford. You accept that you can't do what you once did, and you don't expect yourself to do things that don't work for you. If your partner isn't in this phase yet, they may still be pushing you to do things together that you feel you cannot do. Instead of getting angry about this, try to empathize with their desire to do things with you, and offer alternative ideas for spending time together that will work for the energy you have.

We've talked a lot about fun activities, but keeping up with the household chores and handling other errands are also shared activities. If your partner has not reached this point yet, they may still feel resentful that you're not doing as much, even if you've accepted that your house may not pass the white glove test anymore. Try to empathetically ask what your partner is still unhappy with about the division of labor, and explain that while you've accepted your limitations, you still care about fairness and sharing the load. See if you can brainstorm and test out some ideas for sharing these tasks that fit with your values and energy. But at least convey to your partner that you care about this issue. This'll go better if you can begin by appreciating all your partner has done and is doing. Try saying "I feel like you're doing so much around the house just with things that need to be done. I'm open to sitting down and really negotiating who does what, now that I have different limitations than I used to."

If your partner is the one who has reached testing and acceptance, some of the activities they're doing to take care of themself may not include you. This can feel really bad, especially if you're not in this phase of acceptance yet. Work on compassion for your partner—if they feel calm and balanced in their life, this is only going to be a net positive for you overall. Try to encourage them to continue the things they have found that work for them, even if it hurts you to accept.

Of course, you may still need to advocate for more shared activity as well, or ask to be a part of something that they've found they like doing, even if you can't fully participate. For example, let's say they've joined a running club, which really helps them disperse the stress of caregiving. Perhaps you could wait at a coffee shop near the end of the running route, and when the run is finished, you can have breakfast together. Try to think outside the box in ways that can still support your partner.

EXERCISE: Create a Self-Compassion Journal

This has been a long, hard journey. Take some time to journal your experiences through the different stages and how you've arrived here at temporary acceptance. Make it an actual practice to have self-compassion for yourself. You've been through (and are still going through) one of the most difficult life experiences, and here you are planting yourself firmly in reality. Note the activities you love doing, and allow yourself to enjoy them, even if your partner isn't doing them with you. Have compassion for yourself and your partner if there are activities you can no longer do together. Allow yourself to breathe and observe how you're feeling now, and thank yourself for the hard work that you've done to get here.

Intimacy and Sex

If you're both in testing and acceptance, you've found ways of being sensual and sexual together that work for you and feel good to both of you. Remember that even in partnerships where there is no illness issues, sexual compatibility, style, and frequency change over the lifespan. It's just impossible that whatever you decide today is going to work for both people as you age and as hormones fluctuate and change—even without chronic illness in the picture! Enjoy where you are now, but stay in communication about how things are feeling, and commit to always desiring to be close, even if it looks different from time to time. Being in the testing and acceptance stage with intimacy and sex means that you're committed to having this be a continued part of your connection, you're willing to talk openly about how it's working for you, and you understand that changes are not a bad thing, but to be expected.

Well Partner

If you've arrived at this phase, hopefully you've done more communicating about sex and intimacy than you used to. In this stage you can test out solutions to this issue that may be a little "outside the box" of the sexual behavior that's considered standard for healthy relationships. Again, if you're in this phase, you may have found ways to enjoy sensuality and closeness with your partner outside of intercourse or other activities you used to do, and you may feel satisfied with this new normal. But if your partner isn't in this stage, or if your partner is and you aren't, one of you may still feel unsatisfied in this area. It's okay to feel content with where you are now, even if your partner doesn't—as long as you understand that this is a *joint* activity, so if one of you is unhappy, it's not a done deal. As I've said, try not to feel offended if what is working for you is still not working for your partner. This isn't a statement about your desirability or skill in the sexual realm; it's just that we are all different, and meeting everyone's needs all the time is quite a challenge.

Sick Partner

Hopefully coming to the testing and acceptance stage doesn't mean that you've decided to be okay without any sex or intimacy when in fact deep down you still want it. If that's the case, I beg you to let your partner know this, so that they can make their own choices about how they'll need to take care of their own needs. Your partner is still healthy, so hopefully testing and acceptance for you means that you've identified some sensual and sexual activities that feel good to you, work for you, and do not deplete your energy reserves. Even if you've done a good job doing this, your sexual relationship isn't likely to be anything like it was before you got sick. If your partner isn't in the testing and acceptance phase yet, they may still be pushing you to participate in activities you can't do. Be very honest with them about what you can and cannot do, and make sure to let them know that you still *want* to be physically close but that you may need to negotiate changes.

If your partner has reached this stage and you haven't, they may have adapted to these changes, and that may feel threatening to you. It might feel like they've just resigned themselves to "less than" they really want, and you might feel unsure about this. Talk openly about how your partner feels about where you are sexually, and believe them if they say that the adjustments you've made are okay with them. It's their responsibility to tell you if it's not working for them; it's not your job to dig for information if they're not sharing it. Telling them from time to time "I'm open to hearing about any changes that you'd like to see" can invite them to share.

EXERCISE: Practice Self-Compassion

If you're the partner in the testing and acceptance phase, enjoy the sensual connection you're feeling. If you're experiencing any pushback from your partner for being where you are, offer yourself some self-compassion. Yes, one partner is ill and dealing with a changed reality, but so is the other partner, in often unacknowledged ways. It's a *lot*, and you may have felt overlooked a lot on this journey. Take a moment to have some compassion for yourself for going through what you've gone through and having arrived at a place of calm acceptance. This hasn't been easy. Put your hands on your heart, pause and breathe, and thank yourself for working through these very difficult situations.

If you're still testing out sensual connections, have self-compassion when those activities need to be adjusted. It's okay to have trial-and-error experiences, and you're still worthy of love and affection even in the midst of challenges.

Friends, Family, and Gatekeeping

I hope that being in this stage together means that you've been able to communicate effectively with your friends, family, and doctors that you're accepting of your current reality and are finding ways to live a life you both value, given your circumstances. This might mean that you're really enjoying and having fun with your friends and family again, and that they're adapting as well to your new ways of being. It might also mean that you've developed some firmer boundaries around time spent and activities done with these others. This feels much better if you're doing it as a team. I encourage you to not feel guilty if you're "hunkering down" and spending less time with those outside your circle. This isn't a stable state, and as you cycle back through other stages, you may need to call in more help again. But right now it's fine if you want to lay low and just enjoy each other. Whatever works for you as a team is okay, and it's okay to not feel pressured to do things any differently from whatever you've determined works for you.

If you're in the testing and acceptance phase and your partner isn't, you may feel okay about not going to medical appointments anymore, or you may discontinue helping your partner find new ways of coping. This might feel to your partner like you're giving up, and that may not feel good. Even though you may have landed in testing and acceptance, continue to check in with your partner about what kind of help *they* need from you in whatever stage they are still in.

Well Partner

If one or both of you have reached testing and acceptance, you may feel okay about where you've landed in your life even though this wouldn't have been your preferred path. Friends and family can be problematic here because they may agree with you and be happy you've accepted it, but also think this is a permanent state, so they won't understand when you cycle through other stages again. Or they might not be able to accept where you are, so they continue to bug you to find cures for your partner when you're feeling fine about resting here for a bit. Be clear in communicating with your family and friends about what kind of support you need in this stage, and explain that it's indeed just a stage. You can say "Right now I feel okay about where I'm at with my partner's illness. There is probably more that can be done, and I'm taking a break from that at the moment. I will let you know if I need any help or suggestions."

Sick Partner

Listen, if you've reached the stage of testing and acceptance as a chronically ill person, don't let anyone tell you that you're giving up! You have every right to decide that you're okay with how things are right now and to find your way of honoring your values *however you want to do that.* Your friends and family—and even your doctors—may not understand this and may push you to continue to turn over every rock for a new treatment or cure. It's perfectly okay to tell them that you're pausing for a bit to catch your breath and rest. This is a marathon, not a sprint, and from time to time you need to just pause and recalibrate. Communicate to your friends, family, and doctors that you've found a way to live that works for you right now, that it may not always be the case, and that you'll let them know when to call the cavalry back in. But for right now, you'd appreciate it if they'd just support you in being okay where you are.

EXERCISE: Experiment with Testing

Continue to test new ways of doing things that feel good to you and that match your reality and your available energy. Each time you test a new possibility, make sure that it aligns with your values and life goals, even in the context of your present circumstances. You might want to write down each of your new committed actions and line them up with the values that they correspond with. Remind yourself that this isn't a fixed place, and that life and circumstances can change, but this journal will help you if you end up cycling back through other stages again.

EXERCISE: Set New Goals Based on Values

Write a little bit in a journal about what your reality gap is. What are the things that you want to do, thought you'd be doing, but aren't able to do now? Then try to find acceptance of or perspective on this gap. This may not always be this way, and it might be possible to get back to those things someday. But *today* these things aren't possible for you. Now figure out what values underlie these things that you had wanted to do. What was the meaning behind them? How did that activity represent who you really are inside? See if you can come up with some new, creative solutions for goals and activities that you might do that would also line up with that value *and* be possible the way things are right now, today. Again, things might be different someday, but they are what they are today, so what is possible for you to do today? Lastly, when you engage in pursuing these new goals, you might occasionally feel pangs of regret; remind yourself of the value that underlies these actions and why it's important to you.

Moving On

We have now gone over all of the phases you might experience in chronic illness and some skills you both can use to work your way through these phases, both alone and together. Although a book can't cover every nuance of every entirely unique couple, I hope you can extrapolate some things that are useful to you. We've almost come to the end of our journey, but I want to talk about one more thing in the next chapter—that is, what to do if your partner is hostile to this process or simply uncooperative in taking this journey with you.

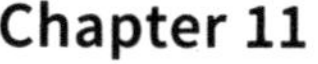

Chapter 11

Going Forward

We're near the end of our journey together. I hope that there has been some value to you and your relationship as we have talked through this process together. This is such a complex issue, because there's so many ways that this may have played out in your life and relationship, and there's just no way to cover every possible iteration of this journey.

I've laid out this process for you in this book in a fairly organized manner, to introduce you to the stages and skills and how they might work together. (See the figure in chapter 1.)

This may be all you need as you go through your process. It may be that the way I've described these stages and skills nicely lines up with your journey, so that in the shock and denial stage, present moment awareness is what makes sense for you. And in the anger stage, maybe cognitive defusion is exactly what you need.

But maybe not! I want you to look at these stages and skills as interchangeable, feeling free to mix and match. For example, you may be in the depression stage, but finding values are really what resonates with you at this point in your experience, rather than self-as-context. That's fine! You can read the first part of the chapter on depression, and then flip to the bargaining chapters for the ACT skill you're looking for. Your experience is entirely your own, and the best way to move through this process is the way that *works for you*. Think of these as two overlapping pie charts or wheels; any stage could match up with any skill if that's the way the process makes sense for you.

The goal of acceptance and commitment therapy is psychological flexibility, and in the spirit of that goal, I extend to you the flexibility of using this model in whatever way that you see fit. This may also change as life happens. Maybe when you're first diagnosed and read this book, you follow the pattern I've laid out exactly. Then maybe ten years down the road you have some issues, and this time the stages and skills don't quite line up the same. All of this is perfectly normal and fine, and you can use these skills in different stages, all at once, or not at all! Whatever works for you is great.

The other concern you might have at this point is what to do if you're reading or have read this book and find it useful but your partner hasn't, or won't participate. What then?

What if My Partner Won't Work This Process?

Lucy was a chef of some renown before the pandemic. Not only was she out of work during the pandemic, but then she got COVID, and it seems like it ruined her life. Lucy never really recovered and is now diagnosed with long COVID and POTS. For a long time, Lucy tried to get into every long COVID clinic and tried every possible remedy. Then she dipped into deep depression. When Lucy started working with me, her partner, Rich, had no interest in coming with her. So Lucy worked on herself alone. She identified some of her values. She can't stand for long enough periods to be a chef anymore, but she started a social media channel with cooking tips, and it's really taken off. She enjoys doing it, and she's able to do it quite often.

Rich, on the other hand, never really came around. He's stuck in the anger stage, partly because he doesn't even believe in long COVID. Rich and Lucy had some differences before the pandemic even hit, and it hasn't gotten better. Rich just rolls his eyes at Lucy's fatigue and is pretty mad that their sex life isn't up to his preferences. They've been living like this for a long time, and it seems like Rich has no interest in making things better. Lucy knows that leaving is an option, but right now, she's covered by Rich's insurance, and some of her treatments wouldn't be possible without it. So she decides to stay and do the best she can. Another of Lucy's values is being loving, so her strategy is just to do what she can do, which is to be loving and kind regardless of how Rich is treating her.

Maldeep was in a car accident several years ago and became a paraplegic. He gets around in his wheelchair but obviously needs a lot of help with many tasks he never used to need help with. Ramona, his wife, isn't having it. She thinks Maldeep drove recklessly in the first place, and why should she have to change her life because he didn't drive carefully? Maldeep tries to negotiate his needs with her, but she isn't interested in helping. Ramona verbally abuses him when he asks her for help, and she refuses to drive him to important doctor appointments. Maldeep loves Ramona, but is clear that he's now in an abusive relationship, and he makes the decision to separate and acquire paid help for what he needs. He's got enough to deal with just coping with his new life, and he can't tolerate abusive behavior while he's doing that.

If your partner is hostile or not interested in healing with you in this process, you basically have a couple of options. For some of you, even after reading this book and defining your values, you may decide that the relationship you're in isn't sustainable for you. If you're the sick partner and your partner does not believe you or support you, or is abusive to you, you must consider leaving the relationship and finding healthier support systems. If you're the well partner, it's okay to consider whether this relationship will continue to work for you now that life has changed so drastically. It's easy for outsiders to look at what's happening and think you'd be a jerk to leave when your partner is disabled. But if you cannot stay and build a life of meaning that lines up with your values, and if you can't be the supportive person your partner needs, it's possible that leaving may be the better option for both of you.

The option I like to try with my clients before those considerations come into play is determining whether you can build a life of value and meaning without your partner's participation. Whatever the state of your relationship was before this illness happened, all of those dynamics are only going to be amplified now. And let's face it, none of us have a perfect relationship! So if this situation has caused you *both* to read this book and get help, bravo! But it may also be that only one of the two has picked up the book or is concerned about how this relationship will work now.

If that's the case, you can still go through this process and see where it gets you. If you're the well partner and you read the sick partner sections—or vice versa—hopefully that has helped you develop some understanding and empathy for your partner's position. That's a great place to start. I do believe that relationships can change one person at a time, and if you become more aware of your own participation in a relationship and clean your own side of the street, things may get better.

Be aware of the phases that you're in, and do your best to practice the things you have power over in these times. Learn the skills that I've explained, and live according to your values *no matter* how your partner is reacting and responding to you. It does take two to fight and be nasty, and it's hard to fight with someone who won't engage in the dispute. Stand up for yourself, of course, but with kindness and integrity so that you can be proud of how you acted regardless of what happens. If the relationship itself does not bring you satisfaction, try to focus on the goals that align with your values and know that you can still build a life you're proud of even if your partner isn't coming along.

Final Thoughts

As I've repeated, there are as many unique circumstances as there are relationships. You may not have found yourself in these pages, exactly. Your anger phase may require "being present" instead of "cognitive defusion." It's okay if the skills and the stages don't line up for you the way I've presented them here. However you need to parse this information together that works for you is fine.

It's not right or fair that this situation has happened to you, but here you are. Chronic illness is, in my opinion, one of the hardest issues my clients deal with—and that's individually! Then you add in the relationship, and things can get complex really quickly. I hope you've found a few tools in these pages that will help make this journey a bit easier for you. Dealing with chronic illness is very much like a grieving process, and grieving isn't fun—at all. There are days when you have the capacity to work through the stages and practice the skills, and there are days when you want to throw this book across the room. All of this is normal.

I've listed some resources in the appendix of this book; I hope those will help as well. Remember that this a very difficult road. Remember to be gentle with one another and with yourselves.

Acknowledgments

Thank you to every one of my chronic illness clients, who have taught me so much about the support that we need and want when we are not well. I have learned so much from each of you, and it's been my honor to support you.

Thank you, Dr. Jacqueline Keedy, for never suggesting my issues were "all in my head," or telling me I was just depressed, anxious, or overweight. There are still heroes in healthcare, and you're one of mine!

My acquiring editor, Georgia Kolias, has believed in every idea I've had, and made my books so much better than I ever could have dreamed through the magic of editing. Thanks for always championing my ideas.

Thank you to Jeannie Wolitzer, Olivia Belknap, and Erin Batali for the help in reading and providing feedback. You're the best kind of colleagues!

To Lisa Herrington for being the best best friend in the world!

Thanks to my husband, Tom, for his tireless support of me throughout my own chronic illness journey, and in every other area of life for over twenty-five years. Here's to twenty-five more, at least!

Resources

Books:

See references.

Websites:

Center for Chronic Illness—http://www.thecenterforchronicillness.org

National Organization for Rare Disorders—http://www.rarediseases.org

Hey Peers—http://www.heypeers.com

The Mighty—http://www.themighty.com

My Good Days—http://www.mygooddays.org

Well Spouse Organization—http://www.wellspouse.org

Podcasts:

The Spoonie Podcast with Emily Fraser

Hope and Help for Fatigue & Chronic Illness with the Institute for Neuro-Immune Medicine

The Chronic Illness Therapists with Destiny Davis

The Chronic Connection Podcast (not running, but past episodes are available)

Emotional Autoimmunity with Kerry Jeffery

Phoenix Helix Podcast with Eileen Laird (not running, but past episodes are available)

References

American Hospital Association. 2007. "Focus on Wellness." *Health for Life* Fall. http://www.aha.org/system/files/content/00-10/071204_H4L_FocusonWellness.pdf.

Bernhard, Toni. 2010. *How To Be Sick: A Buddhist-Inspired Guide for the Chronically Ill and Their Caregivers*. Somerville, MA: Wisdom Publications.

Bernhard, Toni. 2015. *How to Live Well with Chronic Illness and Chronic Pain: A Mindful Guide*. Somerville, MA: Wisdom Publications.

Douthat, Ross. 2021. *The Deep Places: A Memoir of Illness*. New York: Convergent Books.

Dusenbery, Maya. 2018. *Doing Harm: The Truth About How Bad Medicine and Lazy Science Leave Women Dismissed, Misdiagnosed, and Sick*. New York: Harper One.

Fern, Jessica. 2023. *Polywise: A Deeper Dive into Negotiating Open Relationships*. Victoria, BC: Thornapple Press.

Fern, Jessica. 2020. *Polysecure: Attachment, Trauma and Consensual Nonmonogamy*. Victoria, BC: Thornapple Press.

Fogel Mersy, Lauren, and Jennifer A. Vencill. 2023 *Desire: An Inclusive Guide to Navigating Libido Differences in Relationships*. Boston, MA: Beacon Press.

Harris, Russ. 2009. *ACT Made Simple: A Quick-Start Guide to ACT Basics and Beyond*. 2nd ed., revised. Oakland, CA: New Harbinger Publications.

Katie, Byron. 2021. *Loving What Is: Four Questions That Can Change Your Life*. Revised edition. Nevada City, CA: Harmony Books.

Kaufman, Miriam, Cory Silverberg, and Fran Odette. 2007. *The Ultimate Guide to Sex and Disability: For All of Us Who Live with Disabilities, Chronic Pain, and Illness.* Hoboken, NJ: Cleis Press.

O'Rourke, Meghan. 2023. *The Invisible Kingdom: Reimagining Chronic Illness.* New York: Riverhead Press.

Ramey, Sarah. 2020. *The Lady's Handbook for Her Mysterious Illness.* New York: Anchor Books.

Lisa Gray, LMFT, is a licensed mental health professional with a private practice in the San Francisco Bay Area, where she specializes in high-conflict couples and chronic illness/pain. After working as an air traffic controller for ten years, and serving as a peer-debriefing counselor for fellow controllers, Gray decided to go back to school to study counseling. She graduated from John F. Kennedy University in 2004 with a master's degree in clinical counseling, and has been working in the field ever since. Gray is passionate about teaching couples to practice healthy conflict, so that their relationships can thrive and grow. Gray reviews self-help books on her Instagram, Therapy Book Nook. She lives in the Bay Area with her family and three large dogs.

Foreword writer **Cynthia Li, MD,** graduated from The University of Texas Southwestern Medical Center, and has practiced internal medicine in settings as diverse as Kaiser Permanente Medical Center, San Francisco General Hospital, and St. Anthony's Medical Clinic for the homeless. She currently serves on the faculty of the Healer's Art program at the UCSF School of Medicine, and has a private practice in integrative and functional medicine. She lives in Berkeley, CA, with her husband and their two daughters. She is author of *Brave New Medicine*.

Real change *is* possible

For more than fifty years, New Harbinger has published proven-effective self-help books and pioneering workbooks to help readers of all ages and backgrounds improve mental health and well-being, and achieve lasting personal growth. In addition, our spirituality books offer profound guidance for deepening awareness and cultivating healing, self-discovery, and fulfillment.

Founded by psychologist Matthew McKay and Patrick Fanning, New Harbinger is proud to be an independent, employee-owned company. Our books reflect our core values of integrity, innovation, commitment, sustainability, compassion, and trust. Written by leaders in the field and recommended by therapists worldwide, New Harbinger books are practical, accessible, and provide real tools for real change.

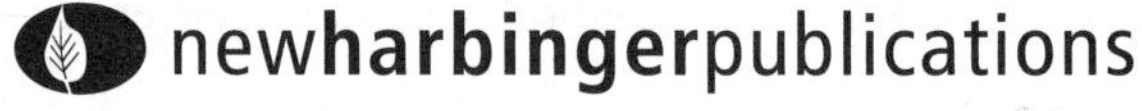

MORE BOOKS from NEW HARBINGER PUBLICATIONS